Praise for
HOMEBREW
VINEGA

"**As scientifically rigorous as it is historically rich.** Kirsten Shockey's elixirs will satisfy curious chefs, home cooks, gardeners, and citizen scientists."
— **DAN BARBER**, chef and co-owner of Blue Hill and Blue Hill at Stone Barns and author of *The Third Plate*

"To call this a fantastically researched, mind-blowingly comprehensive, and very approachable book is an understatement . . . with Kirsten Shockey as your guide **you'll be able to make any vinegar that your mind can dream up.**"
— **JEREMY UMANSKY**, larder master, wild food forager, owner of Larder Delicatessen & Bakery, and coauthor of *Koji Alchemy*

"**This is what was missing from the vinegar world** . . . Kirsten Shockey shows us that there's no limit to what vinegar has to offer."
— **MICHAEL HARLAN TURKELL**, author of *Acid Trip* and host of Heritage Radio Network's *The Food Seen* and Food52's *Burnt Toast*

"Shockey continues her work of helping us understand and **harness the power of fermentation** . . . this book goes into the canon immediately."
— **HARRY ROSENBLUM**, author of *Vinegar Revival* and cofounder of The Brooklyn Kitchen

"Comprehensive and well researched . . . **an approachable guide to the science and magical alchemy of vinegar making.**"
— **SARAH OWENS**, author of *Sourdough*

"**Shockey continues to inspire and amaze** . . . she will teach you how to make quality vinegar but will also fill you with wonder about an ingredient you have taken for granted."
— **MEREDITH LEIGH**, author of *The Ethical Meat Handbook* and *Pure Charcuterie*

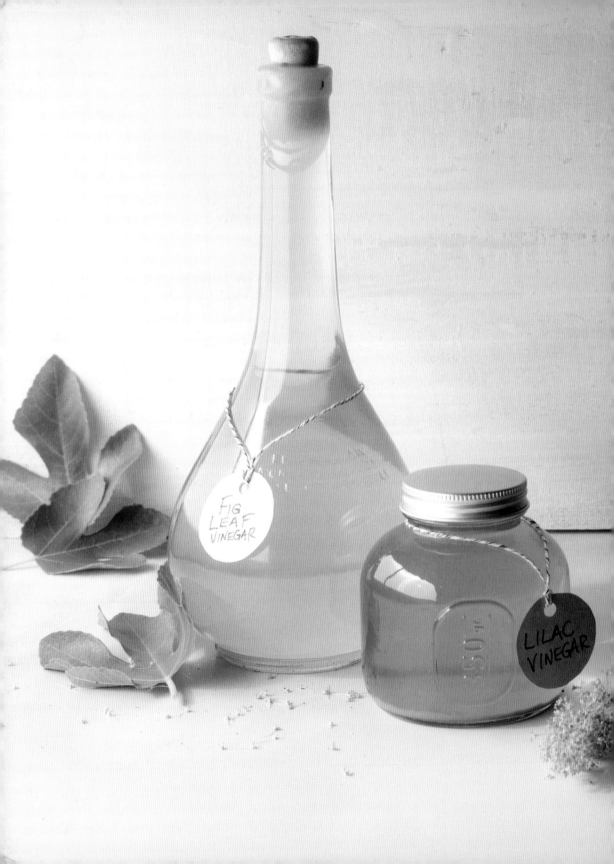

HOMEBREWED VINEGAR

How to Ferment 60 Delicious Varieties

INCLUDING

Carrot-Ginger,
Beet, Brown Banana, Pineapple, Corncob, Honey,
and Apple Cider Vinegar

KIRSTEN K. SHOCKEY

Photography by Carmen Troesser

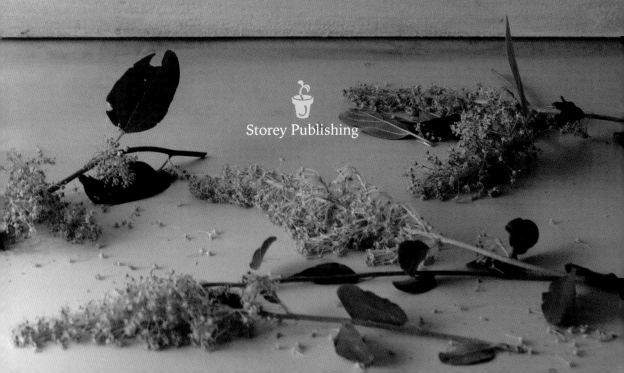

Storey Publishing

*The mission of Storey Publishing is to serve our customers by
publishing practical information that encourages
personal independence in harmony with the environment.*

EDITED BY Carleen Madigan
ART DIRECTION AND BOOK DESIGN BY Carolyn Eckert
TEXT PRODUCTION BY Erin Dawson
INDEXED BY Christine R. Lindemer, Boston Road Communications

COVER AND INTERIOR PHOTOGRAPHY BY © Carmen Troesser
ADDITIONAL INTERIOR PHOTOGRAPHY BY Caroline Attwood/Unsplash, 119; Heather Gill/Unsplash, 208;
J. Rose, Public domain/Wikimedia Commons, 21; Kanō school artist, Public domain/Wikimedia Commons, 18;
© Kirsten K. Shockey, 40, 107 b., 109 b., 271, 274; © Narong KHUEANKAEW/iStock.com
PHOTO STYLING BY Carmen Troesser

TEXT © 2021 BY Kirsten K. Shockey

Storey Publishing
210 MASS MoCA Way
North Adams, MA 01247
storey.com

Printed in China through World Print
10 9 8 7 6 5 4 3 2 1

Library of Congress Cataloging-in-Publication Data
on file

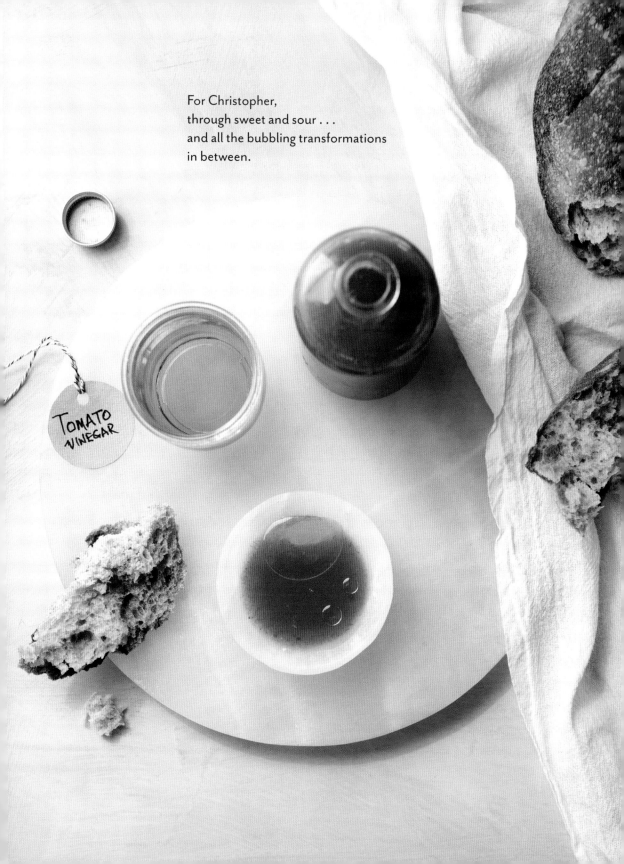

For Christopher,
through sweet and sour . . .
and all the bubbling transformations
in between.

TOMATO VINEGAR

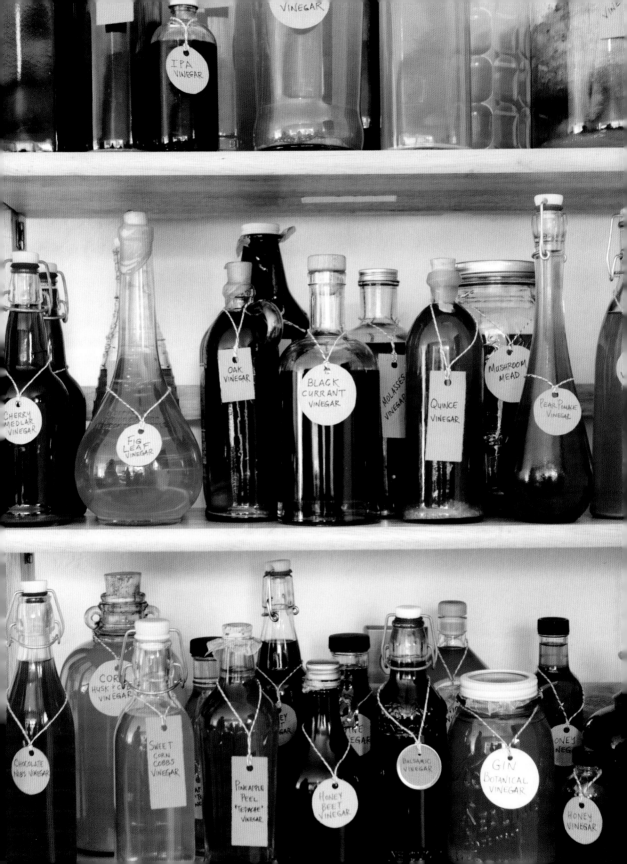

CONTENTS

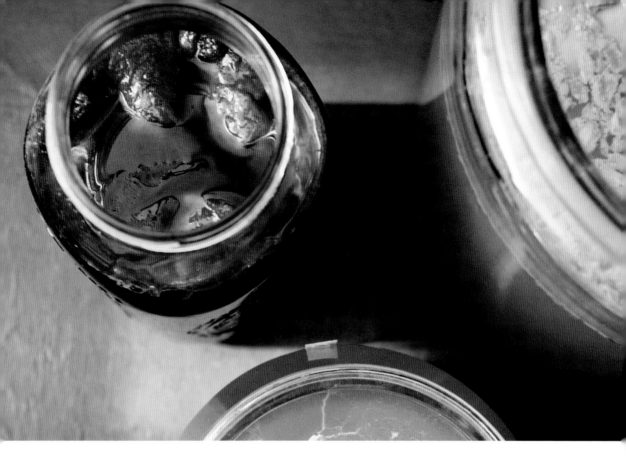

FOREWORD

FERMENTATION, the ancient practice of transforming something raw into something heady and sour, opens up a whole new galaxy of flavor exploration. I am "flavor chaser," so this craft has grabbed me by the heart, soul, and stomach. It has also fed my voracious appetite for knowledge, encouraging me to spiral down wormholes of research, only to emerge with an even more insatiable desire to learn.

In autumn 2014—right before my first book, *Bar Tartine: Techniques and Recipes*, was published—I read *Fermented Vegetables* by Kirsten and Christopher Shockey, flipping from page to page with gusto, exploring untapped flavors and reveling in the Shockeys' playful willingness to experiment. Fermentation is an art of patience and curiosity, and although I had been deep in the maker's mindset for quite some time (Bar Tartine was often dubbed a living larder), the Shockeys became two of my greatest instructors.

The first thing a good teacher does is demystify a subject, or at least ease you in by explaining the basics before building on them. Kirsten teaches this way. With every book she's written, she distills the science into understandable language before applying the theories to practice. There is a gentleness to her style, making new ideas feel approachable and attainable, while arming readers with the confidence and foundation to experiment, so that they can become makers themselves.

How grand is it to let time and terroir transform ingredients into something wholly different and more dynamic than their fresh counterparts?

Kirsten is the type of maker who only comes along once in a while, caring so deeply about her craft that she's spent a lifetime devoted to it. Not only does she fully connect with the process from soil to plate, but she's made it her life's work to catalog, refine, and share fermentation methods so that we, too, can create our own electric and layered flavors. Her first books tilt toward the vegetable world, followed by a deep dive that showed her unwavering curiosity for grains, legumes, and koji. Savory pastes and mind-blowing sauces are the results of such tasty trials. Clearly her larder is as boundless as the craft itself.

So it was with sincere delight that I devoured her latest book, *Homebrewed Vinegar.* Within these pages, Kirsten shares her vast knowledge and love of vinegar, explaining how to make this nose-busting elixir and how to encapsulate flavors within it. Kirsten also explores the ancient wisdom of vinegar as medicine. From shrubs to switchels to oxymels, you're just a sip away from a more balanced self.

Vinegar making, until now, has always felt like a tonic enshrouded in mystery, an indispensable potion deeply revered, yet not fully understood. It is alchemy at its finest; a seemingly magical process of transformation and creation by combining liquid sugar—from juice to honey water—with microbes, oxygen, and time. From there the vinegar is just barely attended to. Instead, it's left to metamorphosize into something more complex and alluring than its building blocks.

Throughout the book, Kirsten takes us on a flavor journey, teaching us how to make vinegar from any number of different ingredients. Thanks to Kristin, my kitchen counter now has a continuous vinegar pot, into which I pour the dregs of wine and cider, and let time do the rest. I've made vacuum-sealed tomato vinegar (page 158), which I use to dress the last of the garden tomatoes and to invigorate winter meals with the whisper and nutrition of summer. I combine lingering food scraps into vinegar jars—their flavor and color lending a lively jolt—while flowers imbue aroma along with offering extra yeast for wild fermentation. Using the techniques outlined in her recipe for wild-fermented floral vinegars (page 124), I've already tucked dahlias from the garden into this year's first batch of apple cider vinegar. And while the wonders of autumn are under way as I write this, I admit I eagerly await spring, so I can infuse vinegars with delicate lilac buds (page 122), the nostalgic scent of my childhood.

If you've ever wanted to learn how to successfully make vinegars at home, this is the guidebook of your dreams. I wish I'd had it as a road map all those years ago when I first started experimenting. After reading this book and following Kirsten's empowering guidance, I can honestly say that I, too, feel more confident in my vinegar-crafting skills. Thank you, Kirsten, for nudging me further down the fermentation rabbit hole. It's a deliciously dizzying path.

—CORTNEY BURNS,
author of *Nourish Me Home* and coauthor of
James Beard Award–winning *Bar Tartine*

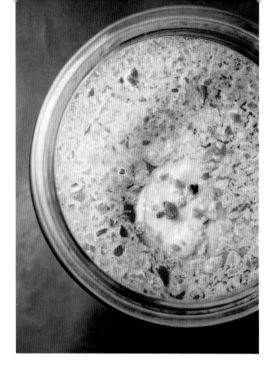
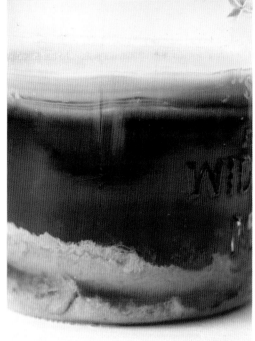

AN INVITATION TO ACID ALCHEMY

WHILE MOST PEOPLE are chasing the perfect sourdough holes and crackling crust, diving deep into the wonders of koji, or just discovering kimchi, vinegar is still one of the largely "undiscovered" and underappreciated members of the fermentation community's bag of tricks. Not to say that there aren't enthusiastic makers, but by and large there hasn't been a strong vinegar movement—yet.

Vinegar making for me has always been an aside to our cider making on the homestead. To be fair, my husband, Christopher, has been the cider maker and I have been the cider taker—or thief, I guess you could say. I prefer "acid alchemist." I shepherd acetic bacteria into both tasty and not as tasty batches of cider and wines to produce the family's vinegar. Vinegar making just felt like an aside—my sour to his sweet— something to build creative tension in our fermentation cave. This book came about in a similar manner. It was conceived of as a chapter

in *The Big Book of Cidermaking*—a very large chapter—one-fifth of the book, in fact. I sheepishly dumped the chapter into the manuscript, and we sent the manuscript off to our editor. A few weeks later, we got an email from her with a subject line of "Can we talk vinegar?" and I knew immediately I'd not pulled the wool over anyone's eyes. The powers that be didn't think cider makers would want a complete guide to cider vinegar, given that most alcohol makers live in terror of acetic bacteria moving into their carboys or barrels.

The apple cider vinegar chapter was pulled from the book and allowed to take wing and explore all the possibility of acid alchemy. As soon as I started talking about vinegar, people started asking questions—turns out there are a lot of closet vinegar makers! By and large, the biggest questions were "Why are my vinegars hit or miss?" and "Why are some so weak that they have to be kept in the fridge?"

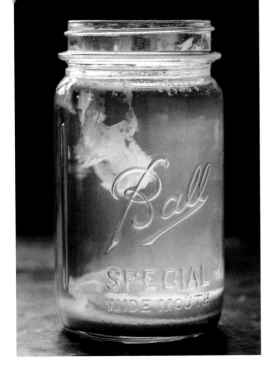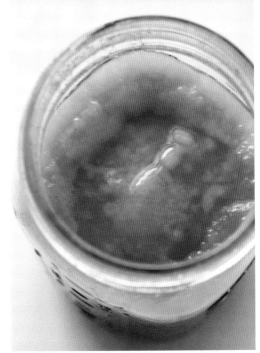

It was then that I realized this book needed to take the path of *Fermented Vegetables*. It needed to become a vinegar class. A class in which you learn how to facilitate, and then trust, the family of microbes we call acetic bacteria. It needed to give you projects that explored the A to Z of anything that could become vinegar—asparagus to wine—and the confidence to go freestyle and make anything you dream up.

Working with microbes, such a fundamental part of our DNA, has been lost and now found. To most of us who have grown up with messages about bad germs dancing in our heads, it is no longer intuitive to let something sit on the counter and transform under the influence of microbes. One fermentation project at a time builds confidence in this new relationship. It's not to say all projects will be great, because they won't. They won't all be tasty, and that's okay because you can always use them as cleaning vinegar. They won't all be right, but luckily when they are wrong, you will know—your five senses will let you know "this is off" (and the troubleshooting section at the end of this book will help). And when you do compost a vinegar project, the soil microbes will know what to do with it. That is the worst that can happen. That's not so bad, is it? Even better, nearly all your projects will blow you away and give you an entirely different perspective on what vinegar is and how delicious it can taste.

You've come to this book with some interest in vinegar. Is it as an alcohol maker? As a fermenter who wants to dive into another adventure with microbes? Maybe you love the power of sour. Or you want to use everything to its fullest potential. Or you are fascinated by the potential health benefits and making your own tonics. Perhaps all of the above. It is my hope that you are inspired to embark on your own journey, or continue on a current one, of collaborating with microbes. I hope you find nuggets that get your creativity flowing and that you innovate your own processes and flavors. Let's do this!

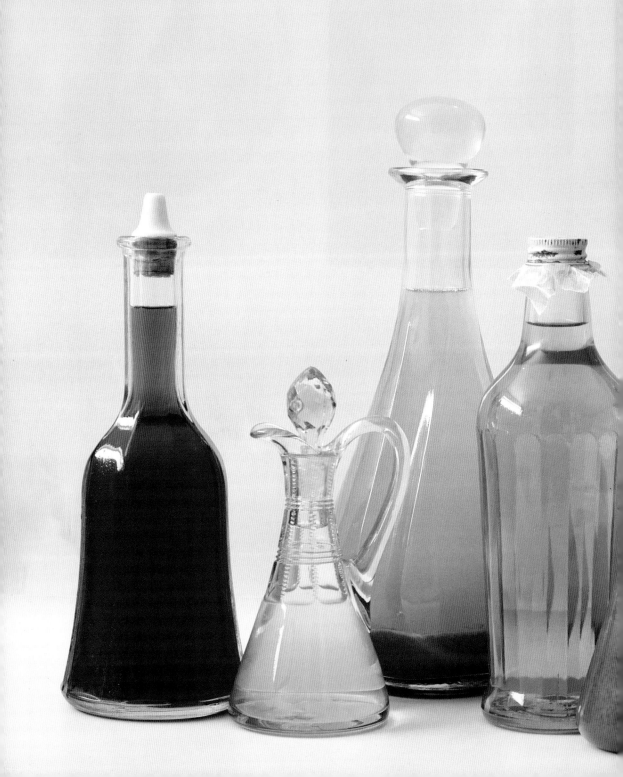

VINEGAR:

You either love it, or you've never given much thought to this ubiquitous sour liquid found in the pantry or under the sink in every household. It comes in two-dollar plastic gallon jugs and in shapely four-ounce bottles that cost upwards of one hundred and fifty bucks. Some folks use vinegar regularly, while others have to dig to the back of their pantry when a recipe calls for it.

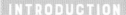

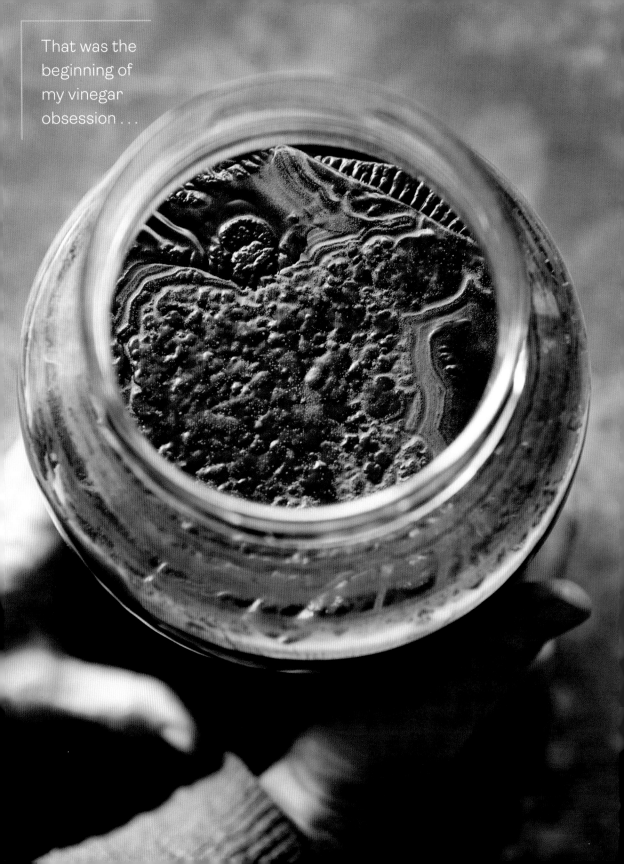

That was the
beginning of
my vinegar
obsession . . .

Because vinegar is generally inexpensive and abundant, people tend to categorize it as either clear, cheap acid or "fancy" red wine vinegar. Simply put, not much thought is given to the wide variety of possibilities when it comes to the flavors of vinegar and what it can be made of. Every region of the world has its own unique alcohol traditions, made from whatever local ingredients are abundant (not just apples and grapes), and where there is booze there is vinegar. Just as each libation has its own flavor profile, each resulting vinegar comprises a combination of unique compounds that impart unique flavors—from subtle to robust. It's time to change the paradigm.

Our son was home recently for a visit and witnessed our houseful of jars, crocks, and barrels all in various stages of fermentation, most of them with the "mother" on top. (This is a peek into what deadline time looks like around here, but I digress.) He asked me, "Why bother? I mean vinegar is tasty, but why?" Although he's definitely in the cider camp with my husband, Christopher, he wasn't asking "Why vinegar instead of cider?" Like many people, he thinks vinegar is cheap and that it all pretty much tastes the same.

I'm sure he was sorry he asked. My eyes lit up, and I took him along for an acid trip through the jars. I dipped a tiny ladle into jars containing vinegar made from fig leaves, IPA, porter, chocolate, turmeric, wild fruits—flavors he never imagined preserved and acidified, ready to add the final sparkle to a dish, like a fine finishing salt. Did I convince him he should try making vinegar? Doubtful. (Let's be honest, though: He doesn't have to any time soon, since he has my larder at his disposal.) But he was blown away by all the flavors and did see that all vinegar doesn't taste the same.

Discovering vinegar fermentation led me down the proverbial rabbit hole, but not right away. The first 10 or so years of making vinegar was just another part of cider making. It was only in the past few years that I realized that, much like in all my other experiences working with microbes, there are methods and traditions to making vinegar. Understand the basics and once you start to play, the field is wide open. You see, anything with fermentable sugar can be made into vinegar (yes, even something like soda pop).

That was the beginning of my vinegar obsession. Sugars are present in so many fruits, vegetables, and grains. (If there is starch, it can be broken down into sugar, which you see in malting and koji making.) I discovered flowers and their wild yeasts could ferment ciders when added to apple juice. Suddenly, the esters and subtle notes of flowers were available, too. The door was blown wide open!

When I started testing recipes for this book, the world of ingredients became unlimited, and it was difficult to know where to stop. Vinegar making is such a universal, versatile way to preserve, and I find the potential is limitless. After teaching you the basics, I've tried to include enough variety of flavors and techniques to give you a tour of what's possible. Some of the most exciting vinegars I've made have started out as "scraps"—peels, pits, overripe fruit, stems, and other items that may otherwise have been thrown away. I want to introduce you to ways you can use vinegar as a tool to turn your home kitchen into a full-utilization kitchen, to minimize food waste. My hope is that you use your experiences to explore your own ingredients and ideas to come up with completely unique vinegars.

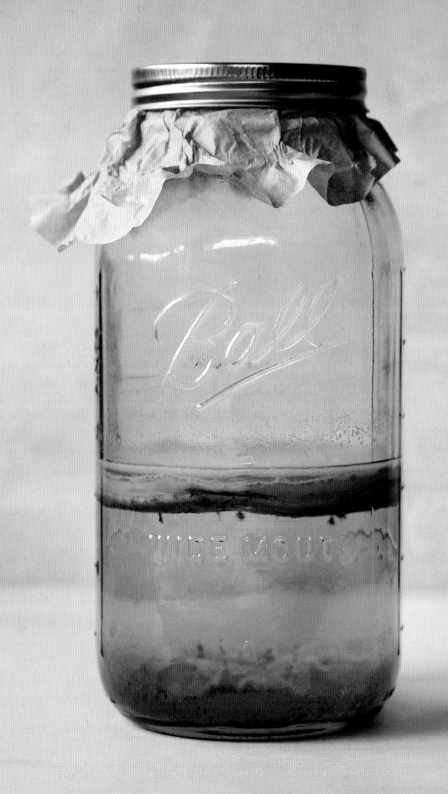

CHAPTER 1

INTRODUCING
VINEGAR

LEGEND HAS IT THAT Hannibal used vinegar to dissolve boulders in his army's path and that Cleopatra dissolved an opulent pearl in vinegar, which she then drank in a lavish move to win a bet with her lover, Antony. But the power of sour we're talking about is all about flavor, food preservation, and digestion. Acidity is an important element in food. The acidity and enzymes in vinegar not only help us digest our meal, but also bring out some flavors while balancing others. Acid brightens foods—giving them a little sparkle on our taste buds, which awaken to all the tastes the meal is delivering. It will enhance a sweet dish by making every bit refreshingly sweet, but will also cut something that is overly sweet. Acid makes the flavor of fats pop as well, and it conveniently washes the oils from those fatty foods off your tongue, so that you will keep tasting the vibrancy of all the flavors, including the subtle ones. In this book, I hope to take you further, to convince you that using vinegar is not just about adding acid to your dish but about creating dishes or drinks that will also showcase the vinegars themselves.

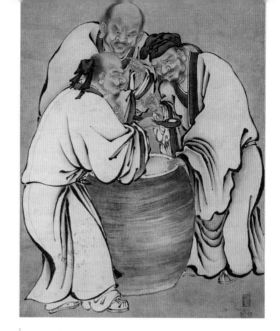

In China, vinegar was listed by Wu Tzu-mu as one of the seven necessities—along with firewood, rice, oil, soybean paste, salt, and tea.

ONE OF OUR OLDEST CONDIMENTS

This simple, universal larder staple happens by way of a two-step fermentation. The process is not complicated, but also not as undemanding as the modern price of distilled white vinegar would lead one to believe. Honest vinegar involves quality inputs and plenty of time.

Vinegar production turned up on the culinary scene along with alcoholic brews, as these two ferments go hand in hand. For thousands of years, vinegar happened in the same way—whether on purpose or by accident—slowly, over time. The history of the word in the West would lead one to believe vinegar is the result of an oversight: The French term *vin aigre* ("sour wine"), which comes from the Latin *vin acer* (also meaning "sour wine"), certainly sounds like wine gone bad. In China, where writings about vinegar appeared more than two thousand years ago, the word *cu* (pronounced *sooh*) is used both for vinegar and as a way to describe feelings of bitterness.

An Essential Ingredient in Ancient Kitchens

Accident or not, vinegar became an essential ingredient everywhere from the humble kitchens of peasants to the palace kitchens of kings. It is central to bringing forth flavor; a splash of acidity will bring life and balance to almost any dish. It has also been an important medicine throughout history and has long held an important role as a way to preserve food. In this book, we'll breeze through many millennia in the history of vinegar in just a few paragraphs, but for a fascinating read looking at the global history of vinegar, you should read *The Eternal*

Condiment: Unearthing the Science, Business, and Sometimes Rollicking Story of Vinegar by Reginald Smith, whom you will also meet on the next page.

Vinegar is a significant staple around the world for all the reasons listed above, and because it is easy to make—it happens on its own with any kind of sugar in a liquid that yeast turns to alcohol. Remnants of Neolithic wine were found in the Zagros Mountains in Iran dating back to 6000 BCE, so we can bet these folks had vinegar then, too. The Babylonians made date vinegar. And according to tomb records from around 1500 BCE, the Egyptians allowed their barley beer to turn sour. At around 1000 BCE, the Babylonians and the Chinese started making vinegar pickles. It is written that Jinyang had large-scale vinegar production in place by 479 BCE, and a vinegar maker could ascend to a prestigious position as the royal vinegar maker. Babylonians also gave us shrub,

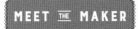

REGINALD SMITH, SUPREME VINEGAR

Reginald Smith is a hobby vinegar maker turned vinegar entrepreneur. His passion for vinegar began innocently enough in 2011 when he came home from Christmas vacation to find that his first home-brewing project—a batch of maple wine—had a vinegar mother on it. Today his company, Supreme Vinegar, is the only supplier I've come across that sells high-quality vinegar mothers to fledgling vinegar makers. The company's website serves as an educational resource for vinegar makers as well. If you find yourself drawn into the world of vinegar, I strongly suggest you read Reginald's blog, *The Eternal Condiment* (see the link on page 285), in which he generously provides a rich source of information, history, and recipes for the "acid curious." (In fact, the kitchen-counter Boerhaave method [page 94] was his idea.)

I originally contacted Reginald when I became curious about vinegar made from whey. Having been a cheese maker, I was intrigued by the idea. In South Tyrol, Austria (think Alpine meadows with big, brown-eyed cows wearing bells), dairy is a staple, and traditional artisan whey vinegar is a delicious amber product. Reginald had recently imported some and sent me a bottle to taste and said he would share some of the yeast.

The sugar in whey is lactose. Like all sugars, it will produce alcohol if you have the right yeast to consume it. This yeast is *Kluyveromyces marxianus,* which Reginald had recently obtained from the USDA Agricultural Research Service Culture Collection. (They will send cultures for free, if you have a company or are associated with a research institution; see Resources, page 285).

My own attempt failed miserably—as in, nothing happened. The whey did not turn into alcohol or go bad. I never knew if it was my mistakes or that the yeast starter had not appreciated the cross-country journey and was DOA. I did a little research, but ultimately didn't have the bandwidth at the time to work it out. When Reginald and I talked later, he said his endeavor had produced a cheesy vinegar.

The positive outcome was that I'd met Reginald and learned a little of his story. His path to artisan vinegar maker and scholar didn't take the straight route from that first accidental maple vinegar, however. Reginald was helping an uncle in Ghana develop and market hot sauce from his farm but realized that there was no domestic source of vinegar. His research led him to Lawrence J. Diggs's vinegar book (see Suggested Reading, page 286) and old industrial production manuals. From this research, he designed a two-gallon vinegar generator with picnic coolers. The hot sauce never became a product, but Reginald was all in. In 2013, he studied with Helge Schmickl, Austrian coauthor of *The Artisanal Vinegar Maker's Handbook*, built his own vinegar generators, and six months later was a small business owner of Supreme Vinegar.

Reginald designed his own equipment and began making vinegar that no one else was producing, using whole foods—mostly fruit or pure fruit syrups. His first product was an ancient flavor: Middle Eastern date vinegar. He continues to seek new flavors. His current interest is in rice vinegars; he's harvesting wild rice to work with. He still sells that original date vinegar, in addition to seasonal and special offerings like rose vinegar, gluten-free malt vinegar, and watermelon and pineapple vinegars, as well as mothers for red and white wine vinegars, malt vinegar, and rice vinegar.

a vinegar-based drink I'll talk more about on page 230.

During China's Tang dynasty (618–907 CE), there were diverse vinegars prepared with ingredients like wheat, rice, and peaches, and infused with kumquat leaves or peach blossoms. Other Asian vinegars were derived from grains and beans—such as the Chinese Shanxi vinegar, which is made from sorghum, wheat bran, peas, and barley. (See more about the process of freeing sugars from grains on page 84.)

As history marched forward, vinegar was mentioned more and more in historical texts for its healing properties. As with other cornerstone flavors, like salt, the acidity that vinegar brought to meals was initially a privilege of the rich (again, it took time and quality inputs). But at some point, this shifted. The poor couldn't afford wine or ales but could have all the soured beverages they wanted—thus it was to become the people's daily drink. Around the same time in China, vinegar was listed by Wu Tzu-mu as one of the seven necessities—along with firewood, rice, oil, soybean paste, salt, and tea.

And so it went for thousands of years; time and microbes converted the alcohol, people waited, and within a few months folks had vinegar. Whether in homes or in fields, where barrels were kept in "vinegar yards," the process was the same: Leave it alone, and if all goes well, vinegar will happen.

The Birth of the Orleans and Boerhaave Methods

In the fourteenth century, wine from the Loire Valley was transported along the Loire River through Orleans on its way to Paris. Any bottles or barrels that had gone bad along the journey were off-loaded in Orleans, so that winemakers could avoid being taxed in Paris for a product that likely wouldn't sell. This was essentially the beginning of commercial vinegar production in Orleans. By October 1394, the vinegar makers organized themselves into a guild; by the sixteenth century, there were more than three hundred vinegar makers in Orleans—all part of an industry that was born by upcycling spoiled wine (something I am happy to report we are coming back to today). Factories there made a slight modification in production methods, which offered more control and shaved off a little time as the wine was being inoculated.

This would become known as the Orleans method (later called the slow method), and it's how most people today make vinegar at home, without the barrels. It involved exposing wine to oxygen over time—usually a minimum of three months. The barrels were arranged in the factory on their sides with holes drilled in them for airflow. To harvest, the maker took out about a quarter of the vinegar in the barrel, leaving behind the mother with the remaining vinegar. New wine (diluted as needed) was put in the barrel with a tube that snaked down under the mother. The downside to the process (besides time) was that the mother would eventually fill the barrels, reducing production.

Producers eventually discovered that finding ways to expose more of the wine to oxygen would significantly cut down the time it took to produce vinegar. One process, described in the journal *Philosophical Transactions of the Royal Society* in 1670, involved moving wine back and forth between two casks with false bottoms

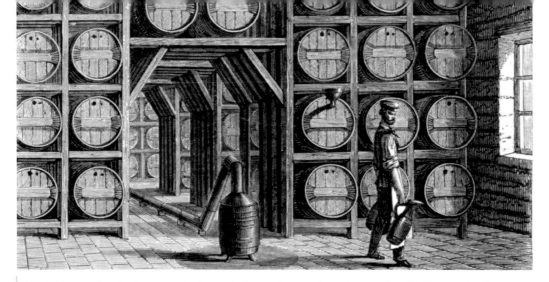

This 1884 engraving of a vinegar-making factory in Orleans, France, shows the centuries-old Orleans method in progress.

that were filled with vine twigs. The twigs were changed daily, as the wine was moved from one cask to the other. In this way, a three-month process was reduced to just three or four weeks. The process was further refined in the eighteenth century by Dutch physician Herman Boerhaave.

All across Europe, makers played with ways to keep the vinegar moving, though it would actually be another century or so before Frenchman Antoine Lavoisier, a prominent chemist, would officially understand that vinegar fermentation can only happen in the presence of oxygen. Finally, in 1873, it was determined that bacteria were responsible for acetic acid production. As soon as folks figured out vinegar was ultimately just water and acetic acid, it was game on for finding cheaper ingredients than wine that would yield more vinegar faster. Heinrich Frings, engineer and son of a vinegar maker, realized early in the twentieth century that there was a market for equipment designed for vinegar plants. Thus, the Frings Acetator was invented in 1954, and vinegar production was no longer limited by exposed surface area. The flavor was compromised, but production doubled. Some systems could even produce vinegars containing 4 to 6 percent acid within a day. The first synthetic vinegar made with wood distillation hit the scene early in the twentieth century.

TASTING AND USING VINEGAR

The secret that vinegar lovers already know is that as soon as you move beyond the basic grocery store apple cider vinegar (ACV) and distilled white vinegar, you'll discover a world of variation in tang, aroma, acidity, sweetness, and bouquet. For those of you who are new to vinegars, I hope to leave you with some hints to take your palate on a journey to discover the many faces of vinegar. As with tasting wine, cider, or any delicious food, you should find the flavors continuing to develop as they linger in your mouth.

What we perceive as flavor is the combination of taste, aroma, and texture. Vinegar's nonvolatile compounds (those that tend not to vaporize) register on your tongue and in your mouth, and its volatile compounds (those that do tend to vaporize) register in your olfactory regions. The tannic combination of astringency and bitterness provides the feeling of texture. All this is sent to the brain, which stitches it together to put words and emotions to what we are tasting.

THE TRUTH ABOUT
DISTILLED WHITE VINEGAR

After speaking with Michael Harlan Turkell, the author of *Acid Trip: Travels in the World of Vinegar*, I came away with a better understanding of what exactly distilled white vinegar is. Michael said "the word *distilled* should tell you so much about what that product is. It is made of a neutral spirit that has no inherent flavor or character." These industrial vinegars, sometimes called spirit vinegars, begin with the cheapest source of alcohol available. Depending on where you are in the world, your distilled vinegar may be made from a base of sugar beets, potatoes, or malted grains. In the United States at the turn of the twentieth century, fermented molasses was distilled for vinegar.

Today, distilled vinegar is made directly from ethanol. Although US regulations require it to be fermented naturally, producers do not have to disclose the source. As you might expect, producers typically use the cheapest source of fermentable sugars available to them—commodity grains, wood cellulose, or even petroleum-based ethanol.

Michael points out that they are making acetic acid, not vinegar. All vinegar contains acetic acid, but not all acetic acid is vinegar. Acetic acid is the main type of acid found in vinegar, typically around 4 to 8 percent. Distilled white vinegars are clear, colorless, diluted forms of the acid. True vinegar, on the other hand, is a combination of acetic acid, water, and other trace chemicals like malic acid, citric acid, and esters that come from the fermentation. All this adds to the unique flavors and aromas that are absent in distilled white vinegar (but are present in white wine vinegar, for example).

The difference between a distilled vinegar intended to be consumed and one that is used for nonedible purposes is a matter of acid percentages, not source ingredients. Legally, in the United States, vinegar must be at least 4 percent acid and no more than 7 percent. At around 10 percent, it's too caustic to consume straight. It can be used for cleaning, however. Horticultural vinegar (also called lawn care vinegar), which is used for killing weeds, is 15 to 30 percent acid. One manufacturer Michael spoke with produced a 5 percent vinegar and a 6 percent vinegar that were labeled as cleaning vinegar; the manufacturer would not reveal the source ingredients for either (which led Michael to believe they weren't food-grade materials).

And yet, pickling recipes far and wide call for distilled white vinegar; I have yet to find a canning or pickling book that doesn't instruct readers to use this flavorless acid to preserve their prime, homegrown produce. Why? Well, it's inexpensive. More important, though, it is clear. People like that clean, clear look of jarred fruits and vegetables, unmarred by cloudy liquid or sediment. Is it that we collectively have gotten so used to seeing a clear pickling medium that a little haze in the jar sends our food spoilage fears into high alert?

The reality is that you can use any vinegar that is over 5 percent acid for pickling. So why not pick one with flavor? You can even have both clarity and flavor, if you want; just choose white wine vinegar, rice vinegar, cane vinegars (see Resources, page 285), or certain coconut vinegars. Your pickles will take on wonderful, complex flavors, and your veggies will not be doused in something incongruent with all the love and care put into them.

When you're tasting vinegar, your senses will first be hit by the acidity. If you stick with it, other flavors will reveal themselves. Getting past the acid can be tricky, as humans have perception thresholds: We don't notice levels of acid until they rise. At the minimum threshold, we can begin to taste the sour (and even like it, as in lemon pie). At the upper end, most of us begin to be repulsed by it or even feel pain.

How to Taste Vinegar

Scientists estimate that 75 to 95 percent of what we taste is actually what we smell.[1] So, tasting begins with smelling. Put a teaspoon or so of the vinegar in a shot glass and let it sit for a moment. Then swirl it around to aerate it. Bring it up to your nose and sniff *gently.* Seriously— take too big a sniff, and the acid can shock your nasal passages. In the first sniff, you will distinguish if the acid is smooth and bright or harsh and burning. Do this twice. On the second sniff, you should discern more subtle aromas that give you hints about what the flavors will be—fruity, woody, smoky, earthy, or floral, for example.

Now it's time to take a small sip. Keep the vinegar in your mouth and let it coat the inside, not just your tongue. At this point, aromas are drifting upward from the back of your mouth to your olfactory bulb, where they are registered and mixed with the smells you already noticed. While the vinegar is in your mouth (don't swallow yet), ask yourself: How does it feel? Your tongue will pick up how the sweetness balances with the acidity (think of balsamic, which is quite sweet with a subtle acidity). You might notice bitter tannins on just your tongue and astringent tannins that cause a puckering feeling on the insides of your cheeks and across your tongue. (These are actually some of the phenolics, page 30.) You might taste some of these flavors in brown rice vinegar or maple syrup vinegar.

The next thing you want to uncover in the flavor is a hint of the base fruit or ingredient. ACV tastes appley, honey vinegar tastes floral and has traces of the honey used, and pear vinegar has poached pear undertones. Molasses vinegar doesn't hide its flavor—it is full-bodied, dark, and sweet, and it screams molasses like a rich gingerbread cookie.

Going beyond Salad Dressing

All this tasting can help you think of how you want to use your vinegars. Acid is a beautiful addition to any dish, as it can affect food in much the same way salt does—enhancing and balancing it. In baking, acid acts in the same way buttermilk does, by adding both lightness and moisture. In savory sauces, it harmonizes the other ingredients (think of homemade aioli). Marinades with acid tenderize meat and cut the fatty mouthfeel. Acids like vinegar are wonderful for deglazing a pan and adding a bright finish to a dish. Homemade vinegars can be used for any manner of quick pickles and chutneys that will marinate and be stored in the fridge.

Talk to any chef, and he or she will tell you that vinegar is indispensable, yet many home cooks don't give it much thought. My job in this book is not to instruct you how to use vinegar in cooking (many chefs have written wonderful books to show you just that—see page 286) but to teach you how to make exciting, delicious vinegars that you will want to splash on everything. I'll also show you how to use them in beverages (Chapter 9) and herbal preparations (Chapter 10). There are so many ways to enjoy flavorful vinegars! Here's to a sweet, sour journey ahead.

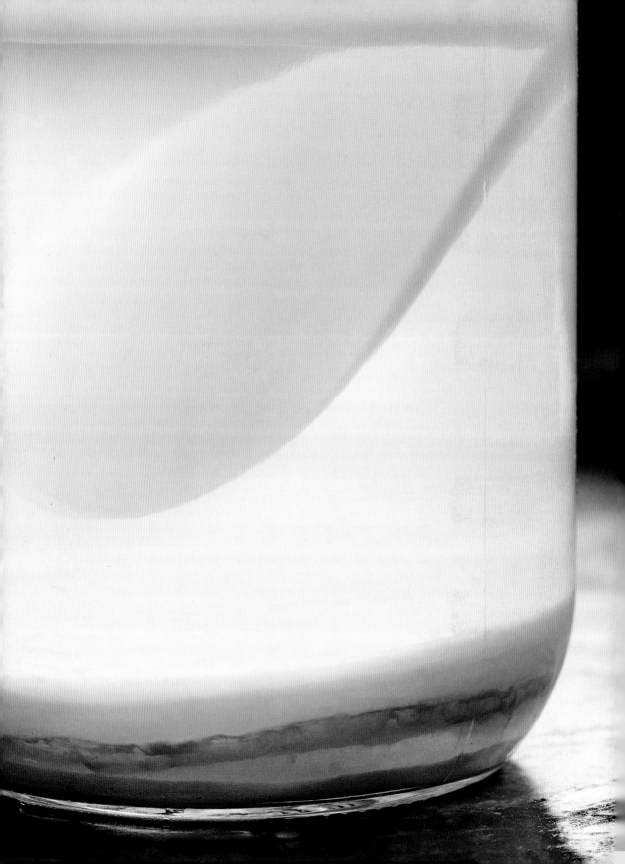

THE
SCIENCE
AND
ALCHEMY
OF VINEGAR

V

INEGAR FERMENTATION RELIES on two microbes that each have something in common with humans (and some might even say our vices): one loves consuming sugar, the other consumes alcohol. When their work is done, we have vinegar. But what is the alchemy going on behind the scenes? What's happening under the mother? For that matter, what *is* the mother and do even we need her? Who are the microbes we're shepherding? Perhaps most important is understanding the acid we're creating and its role in the making of a stable, long-lasting, delicious vinegar.

THE SOUR THAT BEGINS AS SWEET

Once you start looking at fermentation, it becomes clear that it's all about the sugar. Lactic acid bacteria consume the carbohydrates and produce acids as a by-product. Yeast consumes sugar and creates ethyl alcohol as a by-product. This is also called ethanol, though in this book I will simply call it alcohol. Fungi like koji use enzymes to access the sugar trapped in the larger starch molecules, so that they can feed themselves, and we interrupt them because we want to hand the sugar off to yeast or bacteria for other ferments.

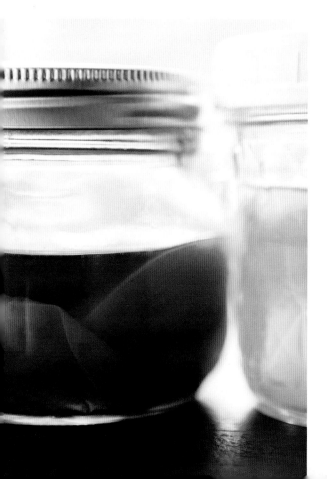

Sugar Turns to Alcohol

Vinegar bacteria go hand in hand with wild yeasts and are also present on sugar-rich organic fruit, roots, and even sap—in short, any fermentable carbohydrate, which yeast will turn into alcohol. In the wild, yeast is present from blossom to fruit; it starts the fermentation that is another step in the decay that begins as soon as the fruit ripens and drops. (And in some cases, before it drops. I often see flocks of birds clustered in madrone trees drunk on late-fall berries.) The sugars increase, and the yeasts begin to form alcohol in the fruit. Time, oxygen, and the warm late-summer sun provide the conditions that wake up the bacteria and start the acidification process. In the wild, alcohol creation and acidification happen simultaneously. In your kitchen, you can make this happen, too; see page 81.

A cider maker, brewer, or winemaker keeps out the bacteria that acidify by maintaining a cool and oxygen-free environment, thereby not waking up the bacteria—after all, nobody wants a libation that tastes like vinegar. In artisanal vinegar works, the fermentation steps are kept separate. The first step is producing a quality alcohol. Only when the alcohol is well developed is it moved to a vinegar barrel or cask. Here the maker provides oxygen and a little warmth, and the vinegar bacteria emerge, consuming the alcohol. Industrially (at the opposite end of an artisan barrel vinegar), vinegar is made with sugar and bacteria as well, though the source of sugar to make alcohol can be synthetic, grain based, or wood based (the tree sugar that is left after the cellulose has been extracted for paper production, not to

Sugar + water + yeast = ethyl alcohol

be confused with the eco-agricultural product called wood vinegar). In these operations, so much oxygen is pumped in, vinegar can be produced in a single day. The more oxygen in the process, the faster it will go. The price is paid in flavor, which is stripped out by the oxygen.

Waking Up the Acetobacters

The terms *acetic bacteria* and *acetobacters* refer to the types of bacteria that produce acid. There is still controversy around the classification as to how many species there are, as they take on many different forms. Therefore, unlike other ferments, in which a pure strain is used (*Bacillus subtilis*, for example, is used to make the bean ferment natto), vinegar is not made from a single strain of bacteria. So you can't purchase a "pure" starter for vinegar as you can for other ferments that begin with a culture, or starter. The starter—whether a live, unpasteurized vinegar or a vinegar mother—passes on a bacterial community that is a mix of different acetic bacteria that originate in a variety of source materials.

Acetic bacteria are obligate aerobes, meaning they need oxygen to live and do not form spores; instead, they duplicate themselves. Also, they have many different levels of environmental tolerance. For example, some bacteria can tolerate alcohol levels as high as 13 percent, while others wither at 6 percent. Some are less tolerant of the very acetic acid that they produce, and die off when acid levels drop. Others can tolerate a much lower pH; they're able to do this by taking the acid into their cell and normalizing (if you can't fight it, join it!). Some species will continue to ferment (or technically oxidize) the acetic acid into carbon dioxide (CO_2) and water. This, of course, will eventually reduce the acidity, rendering it untasty and susceptible to mold. (Given we often don't know the constellation of our bacterial community, this is avoided by removing the mother and bottling for aging. See page 110.)

Generally, acetic bacteria are distinguished by their source (what medium they were grown in), their tolerance to alcohol (something we can

THREE GENERA OF ACETIC ACID BACTERIA

The three main types of bacteria employed in vinegar production—*Acetobacter, Gluconacetobacter,* and *Komagataeibacter*—have different strengths and weaknesses. Combining all of them produces a well-rounded vinegar. In slow production and home vinegar making, *Acetobacter* is dominant. Fruit and other glucose-rich sources bring *Gluconacetobacter* to the jar. Interestingly, this member of the tribe does not form a mother of vinegar (MOV), as it is unable to produce cellulose, like most species of the other two do.

Komagataeibacter, which can survive acid levels above 6 percent, plays a stronger role as acidity increases. Most species involved in modern industrial vinegar production come from this genus.

Ethyl alcohol + oxygen = acetic acid + water + trace acids (+ heat)

relate to), their response to temperature and/or acid level fluctuations, as well as the type of mother they form. Beer vinegar bacteria and a kombucha SCOBY (see page 31), among others, are represented in these wild subgroups. There are also cultivated, fast-acting vinegar bacteria that don't exist in nature. For the purposes of this book, we will focus on cider- and wine-type wild acidifiers and acetic bacteria cultures (the mother).

Acetic acid isn't the only result of the transformation of alcohol into vinegar. Water, other acids, and heat are also in the mix. The heat is something you won't observe when you're making vinegar at home, but it's interesting to know that the chemical reaction of the alcohol turning to vinegar releases heat. The other trace acids and compounds developed in the fermentation are what give us flavors. See page 21 for more about tasting vinegar.

Trace Acids and Esters

Acetic acid is not the only acid in vinegar. Depending on the ingredients used, you will get small amounts of lactic acid, citric acid, tartaric acid, and malic acid. Lactic acid is involved in many ferments, from yogurt to sauerkraut. Lemons and other citrus have citric acid. You've tasted tartaric acid in wine and malic acid in cider and other fruit wines. These will not be forward flavors but will help distinguish the flavors of apple cider vinegar, wine vinegar, blackberry vinegar, or any other vinegar.

Vinegar also contains esters (think big flavor compounds). These are a by-product of the yeast fermentation early on, but they play an important role while the vinegar is aging. They are volatile and continue to change and increase during this aging period, adding flavors and rounding out the sharp edges of the acid.

Residual Alcohol

Acetic acid bacteria imbibe alcohol to create vinegar, resulting in some residual alcohol.

STRAWBERRY OR BURNT RUBBER?

How esters change during fermentation can be unpredictable, and is perceived differently by different people. Strawberry is one example. Its aroma is a complex mix of more than 360 different volatile compounds.[3] Among these are esters, which are the most abundant and responsible for the tasty floral-fruit odors and, in lesser quantities (thankfully), sulfur compounds. Most of these sulfur compounds increase during the final ripening and during biosynthesis (the action of the enzymes during fermentation) and although they are small in number, they can be mighty to the nose—at least for some people. I am one of those people, so for me strawberry wines (and the vinegar they create) smell like burnt rubber. As a result, even though I love fresh strawberries, I don't ferment them.

Believe it or not, you do want a wee bit of alcohol left—0.03 to 0.05 percent alcohol by volume (ABV)—when it is bottled. (Interestingly, most types of vinegar can contain up to 0.05 percent alcohol before they become subject to alcohol regulation. Wine vinegar can contain up to 1 percent.) This is important for a tasty, stable product. (See Storing Vinegar, page 37.) When the alcohol level drops to zero, the same bacteria can start to consume acetic acid instead (because nobody wants the party to be over!). When this happens, the acidity decreases, and the vinegar begins to weaken, gets watery, and overoxidizes. The small bit of alcohol can also help keep the flavor from becoming too astringent or harsh.

As an aside, I've saved some neglected vinegars that had gotten slightly weaker by adding a little bit of gin or vodka. This alcohol boost seems to give the bacteria some food to create more acid and stabilize. This is not a trialed practice, and I don't have ratios as I've done this more from intuition, but it's worked and is something to consider as you experiment.

Although industrial and large-scale artisanal vinegar makers monitor the alcohol level to decide when the party is over, it's not something you as a home maker need to test. For one, it's an expensive process that requires sending a sample to a lab. It's also simply unnecessary. Most makers on the planet throughout history have not tested; they've just learned to identify when the vinegar is done. You will, too. It really is as simple as "Yep, it tastes like vinegar." You will taste sweetness or alcohol in an unfinished vinegar. You will know if it is not acidic enough by its thin, watery flavors; you may taste these when your vinegar wasn't alcoholic enough to produce strong acids to begin with. If you kept a strong vinegar exposed to oxygen for too long and the tasty vinegar has become watery, you will know the residual alcohol is gone.

Phytochemicals

Phytochemicals are chemicals found in plants. Many of them—such as carotenoids, flavonoids, isoflavonoids, and phenolic acid—are antioxidants and benefit our health. They also provide some of the flavors, mouthfeel, aromas, and other sensory qualities in different vinegars. Phytochemicals are especially abundant in fruit

LOOK TO THE PEEL

The highest concentrations of phytochemicals in apples are in the peel,[4] which is another great reason to make scrap vinegar from apple peels (page 192). Likewise, the resveratrol level in grapes is highest in the skins (any red wine vinegar lovers out there?). Like rice vinegars? Studies in Japan revealed that vinegar made from brown rice has high antioxidant activity, especially because of its phenolic content.[5] (The bran is where the magic lies.)

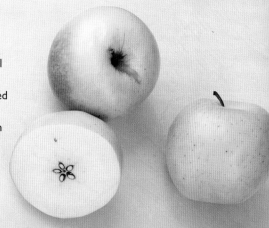

vinegars. The good news is that these phyto-chemicals not only survive both fermentation cycles but also may in part be connected to process-induced transformations in the phenolics and creation of new antioxidative phenolics during fermentation. This means the health benefits not only survive fermentation but can be increased.

ABOUT YOUR MOTHER . . .

The mother of vinegar (MOV) is a superb living organism—or, to be more precise, a community consisting mostly of bacteria and some yeast that has organized into a biofilm. Its Latin name is *Mycoderma aceti*, meaning "skin of the acid." Some of the acetic bacteria species secrete cellulose, which forms this film. This provides the bacteria with a home in which to have

access to oxygen to survive as well as convert the ethanol into acetic acid and water—vinegar. The mother is made primarily of cellulose, similar to what you'd find in plants, just organized a little differently.

It took a while for scientists to figure out what exactly the mother is. In the early nineteenth century, Friedrich Kützing (a German pharmacist, botanist, and phycologist) was the first person to posit the idea that the mother is biological. He thought it was algae and called it a vinegar plant. Then Christian H. Persoon thought it to be a fungus and called it a fungal skin, or mycoderma—fitting given his field was mycology. Renowned microbiologist and chemist Louis Pasteur correctly concluded it was bacterial in 1864. By the end of the same century, Martinus Beijerinck—a Dutch microbiologist

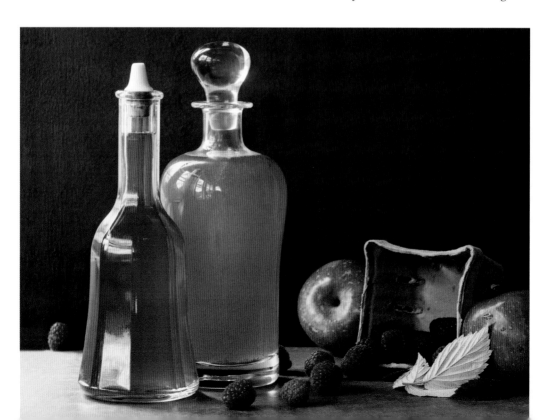

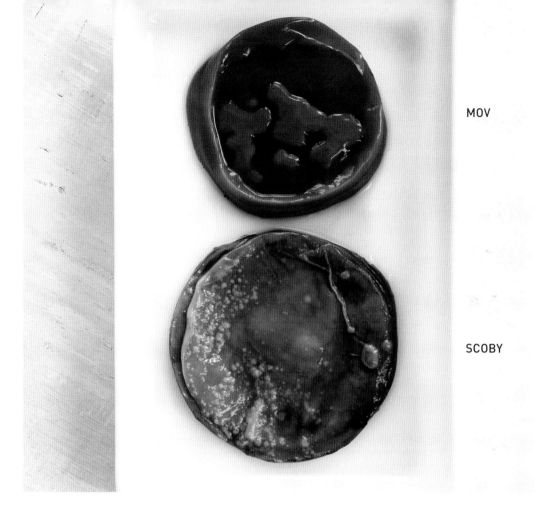

MOV

SCOBY

and botanist, as well as one of the founders of virology who put forth the idea that viruses are infectious—was the first to use the term *acetobacter*.

The strains and variations of vinegar bacteria can cause any given mother to develop differently from another. For example, the mother can look dry, floating on top of the vinegar in progress without becoming wet. As it ages, it doesn't thicken; it stays thin and wrinkled at the surface. A mother can also cover the surface with a layer that looks like liquid; it's thin and makes the forming vinegar beneath it look cloudy. It can also grow up from the bottom of the liquid, looking a bit like seaweed growing from the ocean floor. In my experience, the most common is a film that grows right under the surface. It gets thicker in layers as it ages, just like a kombucha SCOBY does.

MOV or SCOBY?

Speaking of kombucha SCOBY, let's look at the differences between it and a vinegar mother. After all, they both look like khaki-colored jellyfish floating on top of amber liquid. Scientists call both of them a pellicle or zoogleal. Both are technically a symbiotic community of bacteria and yeast (SCOBY), as are kefir grains.

The term *SCOBY* is synonymous with kombucha production and was in fact coined by a booch brewer in the 1990s. The MOV, however, is driven by acetic bacteria and a much, much smaller population of yeast, composed of species that are more resistant to acid. An MOV and a SCOBY can both simultaneously convert sugar to alcohol and then to acid. However, the SCOBY—with its higher yeast content and a lactic acid bacteria community—is better suited for alcohol production. (The resultant alcohol levels are much lower than those of, say, cider or wine, as are the acid levels.) An MOV is usually put into alcohol that has been produced separately by ethanol-producing yeasts that have largely already died off.

A Good Mother Brings the Community Together

Like a good sourdough starter, a good mother brings with it a well-developed synergetic community of bacteria. One study isolated and characterized 96 bacteria from organic and 72 bacteria from conventional apple cider vinegar.[2] (See Is Raw, Unfiltered Vinegar Probiotic? on page 38.) A good mother will have a community of bacteria that is stable at higher temperatures and has a good conversion rate from alcohol: This means it will yield a high amount of acetic acid. In order to do so, the MOV must have bacteria present that are resistant to higher acid concentrations. Finally, those bacteria present don't continue to process the acetic acid and those bacteria that contribute to overoxidation are not present. And as is true with a sourdough starter, generations of people can use the descendants of an initial mother;

the traits of that particular microbial community survive and create the same flavors as the original mother.

An MOV is a satisfying visual validation of your microbial collaborators. It is a confirmation that everyone is there doing their job, and it provides something (someone) to talk to when you're checking in on your project, if you're that kind of person (you know who you are). Another advantage I've found is that a mother on top will slow down the fermentation, so that flavor develops during the fermentation process, not just during aging. It also acts as a lid and seems to keep some of the volatile flavors from evaporating. I noticed this when I was doing vinegar trials, managing the same recipes in different ways.

Do You Need a Mother?

Well, we did to be here, but does your vinegar project? Technically no. Acetic bacteria are in the air, waiting to land on that open vessel of alcohol. The vinegar will happen with or without an MOV or a "backslop" of raw vinegar, because it's a natural process. That said, I prefer to add some previously made vinegar; it will speed up the process and provide extra acidity to ensure a good product. If you ask Michael Harlan Turkell (see page 22), he will say flat out, "Mothers are BS. You can quote me." He feels strongly about breaking that preconception that you need one to make vinegar.

In most cases, an MOV will form whether you want it to or not. (People using vinegar generators find the mother forming in the generator or packing materials to be a nuisance.) A forming mother will be very thin, translucent, and the color of the base medium. If you get close and sniff, you might also get a whiff of what smells like nail-polish remover (acetate). As it grows, it will thicken and look leathery, and may have a white or dusty film of yeast (see page 31). If you let it continue to grow unchecked, it will expand and eat your vinegar. Many of you have likely seen this with a kombucha SCOBY that when ignored for a long time fills the whole jar.

That said, mothers add character. It makes sense that vinegar mothers have the characteristics of the medium that they have been grown on. For example, a beer vinegar mother has specialized itself to convert beer to vinegar. It can be used to make vinegar from something delicate like a perry, but the resultant vinegar will have decidedly malty notes. The good news is that, in my experience, over a generation or two the mother will change and evolve to fit your program. I admit in my vinegar works, I have a rainbow-colored collection of MOVs from the many types of vinegars I make, and they are always floating in enough of their vinegar to keep them submerged and to get a new batch started. I have found that adding extra acid to the mix, especially if the medium doesn't have a low enough pH, keeps the vinegars from developing faults (see page 274) like surface yeast or mold in the early stages.

Backslopping

A common way to start a vinegar is to seed the bacteria, or "backslop" it, by adding raw (unpasteurized) ACV. Many recipes in this book do just that. Do you have to? No, vinegar will happen spontaneously from the microbes in the air, so it is always optional. That said, after years of making vinegar, I find it works quite well, especially when you're working with liquids that may not have a low pH to begin with. Adding around 20 percent of your starting liquid in raw vinegar will increase your success rates and give you less chance of a faulty vinegar. It's the same reason people stick with a good sourdough starter, not starting fresh each time. Any raw, unpasteurized vinegar will work. Until you've made your own batches of vinegar, you'll start with a commercial, unpasteurized, unfiltered apple cider vinegar.

However, since we've been diving a little deeper into the microbial communities that make up the mother, I want to note that the unpasteurized commercial vinegars that most of you will have access to have populations that have been selected for commercial production, which injects oxygen into the production to speed things up. Because these populations are adapted to a high-oxygen environment, using them could cause a batch to start more slowly than if you'd used a well-developed population from a mother, or starter liquid, from your own vinegars.

Choosing to Go Motherless

If you're craving the pure flavor of the fruit medium you're working with, you may want to choose time over efficiency and make vinegar without adding a mother. In most, but not all, cases a mother will develop on its own; it just takes a while. How long? As with most types of fermentation, the answer is "it depends." A mother can take as little time as a couple of weeks to form or as long as a couple of months. It depends on the bacteria type, the type of alcohol and the nutrients available in it, the temperature at which you're fermenting, how much oxygen it's receiving, and so on.

I've made batches that never developed a mother at all but still produced a successful, delicious vinegar. The microbes don't need the pellicle to function. Don't take it personally. I only say this because when a mother doesn't form, it can feel disappointing for some people. If I've learned nothing else over the years of collaborating with microbes, it's that the more I think I understand, the less I do. (Rather like raising children . . .)

In other words, we can only set up the conditions and pretend we are in control, but we are not—the microbes are. Understanding their needs, and stepping aside for them to flourish and create, is part of the joy of fermentation. Of course, sometimes these microbial teams produce things that just don't quite work out like we'd planned. Vinegar is no exception. Having a ferment with a mother, a visual to look at and watch grow, is very satisfying, compared to those where you don't have a tangible long-lived partner in crime.

How Much Mother Do You Need?

Again, technically you only need good-quality raw vinegar to start your own batch. Having a mother can help kick-start it. I asked Reginald Smith, who uses and sells vinegar mothers, his thoughts. "True, you don't need a mother but you don't need brewing yeast either. It is still helpful to have a honed product that is more likely to succeed. Wild fermentation can be hit or miss. The biggest misconception about the mother is the size of solid material. You want some solids but the amount isn't that big of a deal. It is all bacteria in the raw vinegar anyway that should multiply rapidly and form a new mother. Having a one-ounce glob doesn't really speed this up as much as some think."

When I have a mother, I like to start with a piece that covers around one-third of the surface area of the new liquid and the vinegar it was stored with. The larger the surface is, the better results we have at keeping it floating. Ideally, you will be able to place it carefully so that it will float. Thick ones will sink. You can add the mother anytime during the fermentation or to finished alcohol. However, if you are going through the whole fermentation, the best time to add it is a few days into the active yeast fermentation; all that bubbling CO_2 will push it up, keeping it on top. That said, it's okay if it sinks. If it's floating, we don't disturb it, as it is getting the oxygen it needs to thrive and help produce more vinegar bacteria. However, if your mother sinks, it can be a good idea to stir the young vinegar vigorously every day or two to pull the mother to the top and put a little oxygen into mix; this will encourage the vinegar production. If you're hoping a new mother will form, after a few weeks stop stirring so that the biofilm can develop. A new mother usually forms in three or four weeks. The sunken mothers go into stasis in storage, but they can also die. You will know this happened if it turns dark brown. Pull it out when you see this.

To start a vinegar without a mother, backslop with 20 percent vinegar based on the amount of liquid you're starting with. So, for example, if you have a gallon of alcohol, you'll add 20 percent of that volume to it in unpasteurized vinegar, which is about 3¼ cups (769 mL).

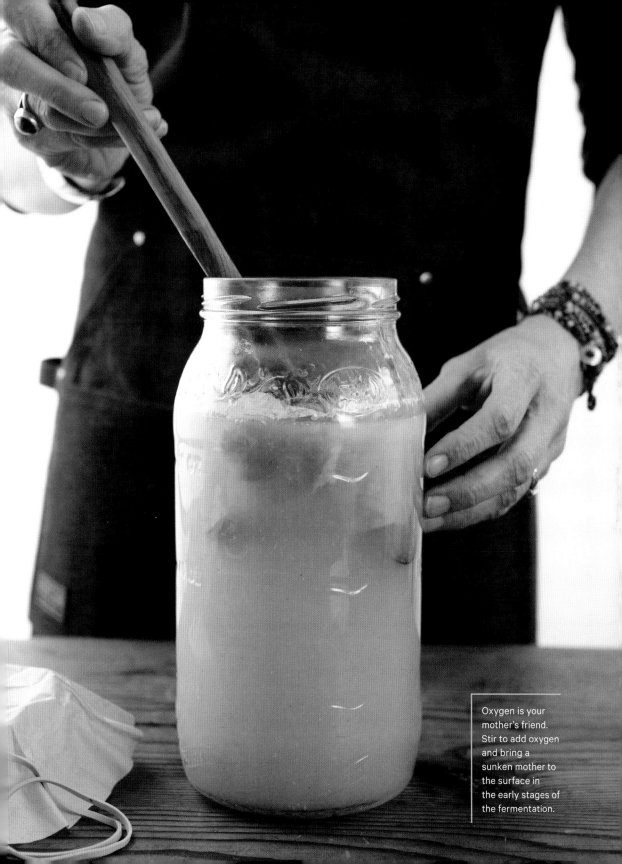

Oxygen is your mother's friend. Stir to add oxygen and bring a sunken mother to the surface in the early stages of the fermentation.

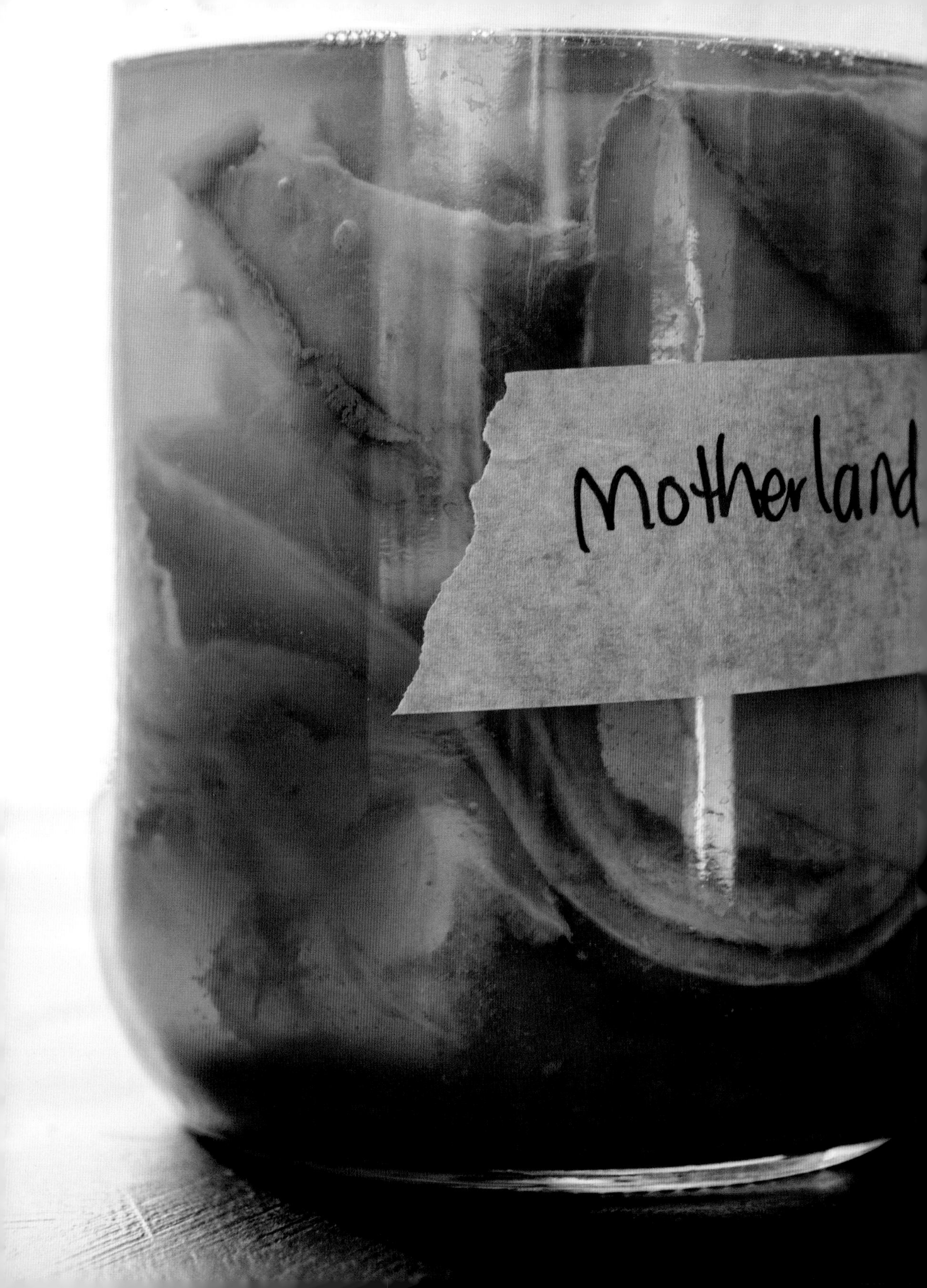
Motherland

Sharing and Storing an MOV

Once you've made vinegar, you will most likely have a mother. You can use this immediately in another batch, or you can use some and divide off a layer or two to share with a friend, or you can store it for many years. (I won't go so far as to say "indefinitely," but I have revived a mother that waited patiently in a jar for seven years, and it worked!) There are only a few rules. Keep the mother fully immersed in vinegar, in an airtight container; you can even fold it into a small jar with a good seal. That way, you won't need as much vinegar to keep it submerged. The vinegar will keep your mother from drying out and becoming susceptible to mold, and the lack of available oxygen will halt any fermentation, in a sense putting the mother into stasis. Storing it in a cool, dark cabinet is a good idea, but honestly the mother-in-waiting is fairly tolerant and can take temperatures up to 138°F/59°C and down near freezing (don't freeze it, though). If you're using a glass mason jar, be sure to place a piece of parchment paper, waxed paper, waxed cotton, or plastic wrap between the metal lid and the contents of the jar; if using a plastic lid, be sure that you've added a silicone sealing ring, as the standard lids are not airtight.

Storing Vinegar

Vinegar can last indefinitely, especially if you keep it out of constant bright light (colored bottles help with this) and high temperatures. Most important, though, keep it in an airtight container; as I mentioned earlier in the chapter, vinegar can overoxidize, resulting in a watery, weak product. Make sure your bottles are always airtight, and transfer leftover vinegar to smaller

ACID PERCENTAGES OF VARIOUS VINEGARS

2.8% Wine Vinegar

3.5% ACV

5%–8% Pickling Vinegars

6% Pure Balsamic

bottles to minimize air contact. You will read more about good bottling choices in Worthy Bottles on page 108.

Keep in mind that low-acid vinegars, such as those made with fruit and vegetable scraps (see Chapter 7), are less stable (the acid is the preservative, after all). These mellow vinegars generally don't need the same amount of aging time, but they also need special storage considerations. They should be stored in airtight containers in the fridge and used within a year to keep them from going funky, or off. If you suspect any vinegar is off, you know what to do—pour it on a compost pile.

MEASURING ACIDITY

It might be surprising, but as you go through the process of making vinegar, you'll find that keeping an eye on the pH can be helpful. You will learn there are two types of acid measurements. The acidity of your vinegar is significant not just in the end product, where one would expect, but also in starting the batch. A higher acidity is important for preservation and protection during fermentation. This low pH will

IS RAW, UNFILTERED VINEGAR PROBIOTIC?

From traditional media outlets to bloggers, anybody who has anything to say about health has something to say about the benefits of probiotics. The word literally translates to "*for life.*"

Probiotics are defined by the Food and Agriculture Organization of the United Nations and World Health Organization as "live microorganisms that, when administered in adequate amounts, confer a health benefit on the host." (For the purposes of this book we're going to assume that's us—human beings.)

Prebiotics are different because they aren't types of microorganisms but rather things that can be utilized by microorganisms. The International Scientific Association for Probiotics and Prebiotics defines prebiotics as "a substrate that is selectively utilized by host microorganisms conferring a health benefit." You can think of probiotics as the live microbes that provide us with health benefits and prebiotics as the food that they select to fuel their work. (*Synbiotic*, by the way, a riff on *synergy* and *biotics*, refers to the presence of both probiotics and prebiotics, usually within a type of food or a supplement.)

Depending on what you made your vinegar with, it probably contains prebiotics. For example, apple cider vinegar (page 117) contains the pectin from the apples, which is a carbohydrate that feeds resident healthy bacteria in our bodies.

Vinegar does not contain probiotics as defined above, because acetic bacteria need oxygen and don't live in our human guts. (If you are a fruit fly, vinegar is absolutely probiotic.) However, much of the current understanding of our relationship with live microbial foods is evolving daily. We now understand that the dead microbe bodies (called postbiotics, but officially known as nonviable microbial cells) also influence the health of our microbiome through the by-products they release. Vinegar does offer this benefit.

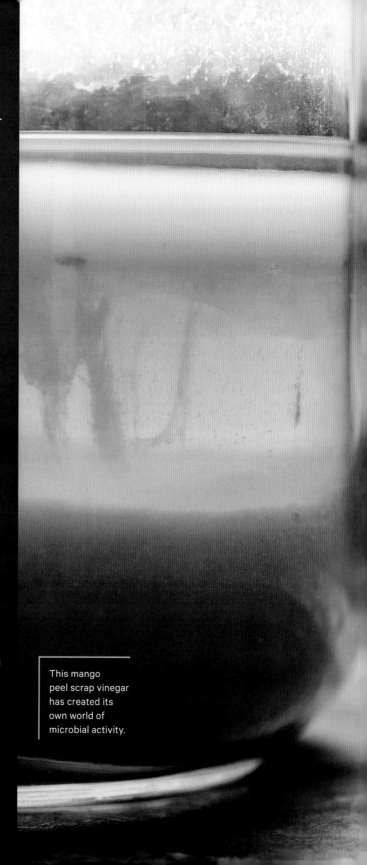

This mango peel scrap vinegar has created its own world of microbial activity.

help keep surface yeasts or mold from forming. This is another reason why raw vinegar is added in the slow processes that are used in this book. Each alcohol comes in at a different acidity, based on the ingredients used. For example, apples and grapes are already quite acidic, so the cider or wine going into the vinegar has a much higher acid starting point than, for example, beer does.

Acid Percentage and pH

Once the vinegar fermentation is finished, there are two acidity measurements to consider: percent acid and pH level. You don't really need to measure either of these to make a safe vinegar for flavor and enjoyment. However, measuring pH can give you a sense of doneness based on acidity; the range for apple cider vinegar averages around pH 3.0 to 3.5 but can be as high as 4.0. To be considered safe from spoilage or other unwanted microbes a minimum pH of 4.0 should be achieved. Ideally your vinegar will come in at 3.7 or below. (If you decide to sell your vinegar, consult the regulations laid out by the Food and Drug Administration and your local health department.) Wine vinegar averages 2.8. But your taste will let you know when your vinegar is balanced and delicious, and that is the point. It's more important to know the percent acid if you'll be using your vinegar for food preservation (see right).

PERCENT ACID. This is the number of grams of acetic acid per 100 mL of vinegar. In other words, it measures the acid content; for example, 100 mL of 5 percent vinegar has 5 grams of acetic acid. (This shows you that vinegar is composed mostly of water.) You may

see the word *grain* describing the acidity of commercial vinegar. By this scale, 10 grain is 1 percent acid, so the standard 5 percent vinegar is 50 grain vinegar. (Incidentally, if this grain measurement were more common, it would take away a bit of confusion around the two acid measurements.)

ACIDITY LEVEL OR PH. The acidity of a vinegar, or the strength of its acid, is measured on the pH (power of hydrogen) scale. This is the one most brewers and food preservers are familiar with. It measures the concentration of hydrogen ions to determine the acidity or alkalinity of a substance. The scale ranges from 0 to 14, with 7 being neutral (water is generally right around 7). Both acidity measurements have their place but are not interchangeable; there is not a pH measurement that corresponds with a percent acid. The reason for that is because different varieties of vinegars that may all have the same percent acid may have varying pH qualities based on the base fruit and the compounds it brings to the table. While pH is easy to measure with simple pH litmus strips or a pH meter, measuring percent acid is a titration process. (See Home Titration, page 42.) And this is where the home maker can get confused.

Vinegar for Food Preservation

It's important to know the percent acid if you'll be using your vinegar for preserving food through canning or pickling. Vinegar must be at least 5 percent acid for these activities, which is what most commercial vinegar in North America is. For perspective, most table vinegars range from 3.5 to 7 percent. Traditional balsamic of Modena and wine vinegar are both around

A TOUR OF
HIGH-ACID
VINEGARS

MANY PEOPLE MAY not be aware that vinegar can come in very high concentrations of acid. In some areas of the world, these inhabit a normal spot in the pantry (and sometimes the medicine cabinet).

The first time I saw a high-acid vinegar, a whopping 25 percent acid, I was on the tiny island of Ambon, in the Moluccan archipelago within the larger Indonesian archipelago. Forty-four years after living in a small village there as a child, I had the privilege of spending time cooking with the woman who'd been my best friend then, Tuti. We went to the market and piled on fresh fish, turmeric root, chiles, sago, shallots, and papaya flowers. With our bags filled with vibrant colors, Tuti then picked up a small plastic bottle with a dropper top and a clear liquid inside. I had no idea what it was. It turned out to be concentrated vinegar, or, more appropriately, a diluted acetic acid. Tuti used just a few drops in one of the dishes.

There are a few areas in the world that have a strong tradition of using these high-acid products for their pickling. Like all vinegar preserving, the tradition started in the early twentieth century with the beginning of the vinegar industry. In Swedish cuisine—which has a strong pickling tradition, from herring to vegetables (it is a long, cold winter, after all)—they use a 12 percent *ättiksprit* or 24 percent pure *ättika*. These are distilled white vinegars. The traditional ratio for using the 12 percent *ättiksprit* is 1:2:3—one part vinegar to two parts sugar to three parts water. This, of course, changes dramatically with the more common 5 percent vinegar.

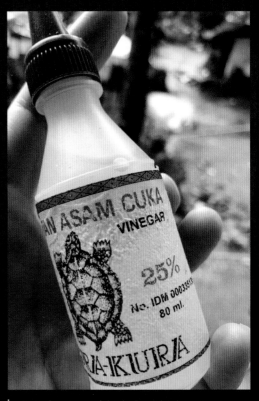

Just a few drops of this high-acid Indonesian vinegar are added to dishes.

One hundred percent *glacial acetic acid*, meaning water-free acetic acid coming from the icelike crystals that form at 61.9°F/16.6°C, is made in a hermetically sealed system to capture the water vapor that is taken out predistillation. The medical industry uses acetic acid as well. For example, in World War II, a 50 percent solution was used for dressing wounds in the field.

In some parts of the world, vinegar contains as much as 25 percent acid.

6 percent, though some of the grocery store balsamics (not the traditional long-aged ones) are around 4 percent, because of added sugar and grape juice. Under 4 percent, the vinegar acidity and subtle flavors get lost in cooking but are perfect for adding to bubbly water for drinking (and may need to be refrigerated for stability). Anything over 8 percent is too strong for most cooking applications. Pickling vinegars are 5 to 10 percent acid. If you aren't measuring percent acid, don't use your homemade vinegars for long-term storage preservations. You can use them for quick pickles and refrigerator pickles. If you decide to go into the vinegar business and sell it legally, it must exceed 4 percent acid. (You will want to take it to a food lab for testing.) If there is an upper limit, I have not found it specified in the United States; in the European Union, wine vinegar is capped at 10 percent acid.

STARTING WITH FINISHED ALCOHOL

Acetic bacteria feed on alcohol, so it makes sense that the percent acid in vinegar can be predicted by the alcohol by volume (ABV) measurement of the alcohol you're starting with. For example, if the ABV is 5 to 6 percent, you will likely end up with a vinegar that has 5 percent acidity. A higher ABV will give you a higher acidity—but there are limits. Since the acetic bacteria will die at about 9 to 10 percent ABV, base alcohol that is this strong must first be diluted. Certain commercial processes can be employed to make vinegar from higher ABV alcohol, but for the traditional slow methods in this book, you will be limited by the abilities of

the microbes and their alcohol preferences. Just as you can get a sense of the ABV of your future alcohol by measuring the sugars in the juice by means of specific gravity (see page 57), this same measurement will give you the potential acidity level of your future vinegar.

Once you've chosen a type of alcohol, there are a few things you may need to do to prepare it. If you're starting with a high-ABV alcohol, you may need to dilute it. If your ABV is low, you'll need to add alcohol. And if you're using purchased alcohol that's been treated with sulfites, you'll need to remove them.

Adjust ABV

Given the preferences of the acetic bacteria that will be turning your alcohol into vinegar, you'll need to start with alcohol in the 5 to 9 percent ABV range. If you're using purchased wine, cider, beer, or other types of alcohols, the label will tell you the ABV. If you've made your own alcohol, use your initial and final specific gravity readings to determine your final ABV.

DILUTING. If your ABV is greater than 9 percent, you'll need to dilute the alcohol. In the case of wines, meads, sakes, beers, and ciders that are higher in ABV, simply adding fresh,

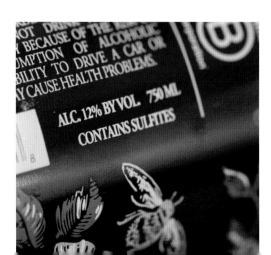

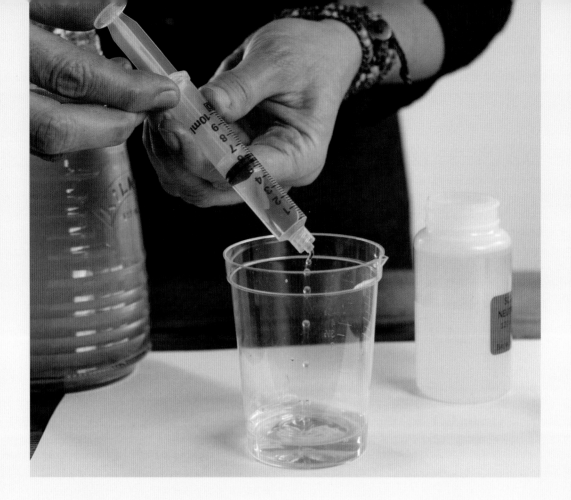

HOME TITRATION

Remember that chemistry set you dreamed of getting when you were a child? Well, if you didn't get one, you can treat yourself to a titration kit. The one I have was inexpensive at our local brewing supply store.

Titration can feel like an overwhelming leap, but like most things, if you dive in you will build the skill and confidence. If you decide to do this, the kit will have instructions, but here is an idea of what to expect.

An acid-testing kit will have some form of these items. Mine contains the following items.

- 12 cc plastic syringe
- test vial
- eyedropper
- 120 mL sodium hydroxide solution
- 15 mL phenolphthalein indicator—1.0%

Titration involves adding a few drops of phenolphthalein to 15 cc of your vinegar. This is followed by the addition of a sodium hydroxide solution to see a color shift in the vinegar. You should work over a white sheet of paper. For the process, you will measure the amount of sodium hydroxide needed to create a neutral solution; this is the color change. The amount of solution added determines the amount of acid in your vinegar. Each cc of solution is 0.10 percent acid, so, for example, 6 drops means the vinegar contains 0.6 percent acid.

unchlorinated water will do the trick. Let's say your alcohol is 14 percent and you want to knock that back to about 9 percent. You will divide the smaller target number by the current measurement. When you divide 9 percent by 14 percent, you get roughly 64 percent. This would be the amount of the alcohol you're diluting, and the other 36 percent would be the amount of water you would add. For example, if you've got 1 gallon (64 ounces) of 14 percent alcohol, and you want to knock it back to 9 percent, you would add 23 ounces of water (64 × 0.36).

You can also work off of approximates. For an average wine, you will use one part water for every three parts wine. For an 80 proof distillate, you will add water at a ratio of five parts water to one part distilled liquor.

In most cases, the additional water doesn't dilute the final vinegar flavor enough to be noticeable. If it is a delicately flavored alcohol, you might take this into consideration and try to build the vinegar slowly with the continuous-brew method (see page 90). With this method, once you've produced the initial vinegar, you start removing some vinegar and adding more alcohol. This is also a way to produce a vinegar with higher acidity, if you're starting with a high-ABV alcohol. Because it's added in smaller amounts, the alcohol becomes diluted in the brew and won't deter the bacteria. If you are already a brewer, you can think of it like chaptalization, where you add sugar in stages to increase the alcohol content.

ADDING ALCOHOL. If your alcohol does not have at least 5 percent acid, you'll want to add some alcohol, such as a clear flavorless 80 proof vodka. For every 1 percent ABV you need to increase, add 30 mL of 80 proof alcohol per quart. This works out to roughly five parts water to one part spirits. This can be very helpful when your brew doesn't quite hit the alcohol levels you need, because the sugar levels aren't high enough in your base ingredients. The recipes in this book solve this by adding sugar in the beginning of the process, but adding alcohol is another way to work with ingredients that won't produce a high level of alcohol on their own.

You can also incorporate vodka or other spirits in vegetable juices to bypass fermenting those juices with sugar (see the Carrot-Ginger Vinegar recipe on page 141). When using the spirits as part of a mostly fresh fruit or vegetable ferment, you can use the slow fermentation method. It is important to note that bacteria still need some nutrients. (I suspect this nutrient need is where the Italian folk tradition of adding a piece of pasta to a vinegar project came from.) If you're using just distilled spirits, you'll need to add a little something for nutrients. Think of it as bacteria vitamins. This could be as simple as a few tablespoons of wine or beer. Because of the small amount of nutrients, you will also need to use an aeration method (page 93) to turn the vinegar before the bacteria run out of nutrients. I have found that with the slow methods, spirit-based vinegars can mold and go bad before converting.

Remove Sulfites

The sulfites or sulfur dioxide that is sometimes added to alcohol can prevent the vinegar from fermenting. Sulfites function as a preservative, which by its nature keeps bacteria from breaking things down. If you want to make vinegar

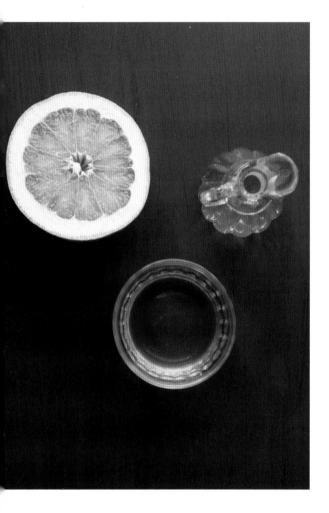

with a product that contains sulfites, you'll need to remove them. This can be done one of two ways. The first is through aeration—either by vigorously stirring to mix in a lot of air or by putting in a small aquarium pump operating at the rate of one hour per gallon (3.8 L). The second option is to add ½ teaspoon (1 mL) of food-grade hydrogen peroxide per gallon (3.8 L) of alcohol. The hydrogen peroxide oxidizes the sulfites, turning them into hydrogen sulfate.

Good Ingredients = Good Vinegar
Good alcohol makes good vinegar. Even though the vinegar makers in Orleans, France, built their factories on spoiled wine, in reality you want to choose solid wines, meads, beers, ciders, sakes, or distillates. For the most part, making vinegar isn't just a way to fix a spoiled brew. If you're a brewer, you know there are variations of a bad batch. Many a nondrinkable batch has become a lovely vinegar. So it might be worth a try to salvage the batch. However, a bacterially or otherwise infected batch will likely stay infected. Vinegar suffers from the reputation of being a mishap or a brew gone bad, but in reality, vinegar is another high-quality ferment that starts with high-quality ingredients.

ABV: "ALCOHOL BY VOLUME" OR "APPROXIMATE BUT VARIABLE"

One caveat that most brewers and makers already know: The ABV percentage on the label isn't necessarily correct. That's because there is some wiggle room in the law to accommodate small craft makers who have some variability in their batches. Tracking the amount of sugar through fermentation (see Measuring Specific Gravity, page 58) gives the maker a good idea of the final ABV percentage, but it's not perfect. The actual ABV doesn't vary by much—less than 2 percent—but you should be aware of it.

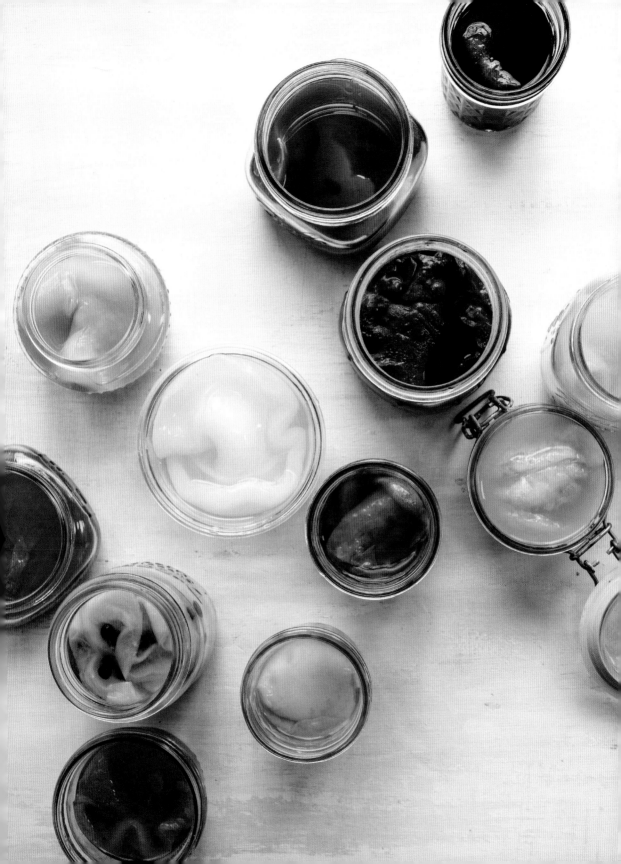

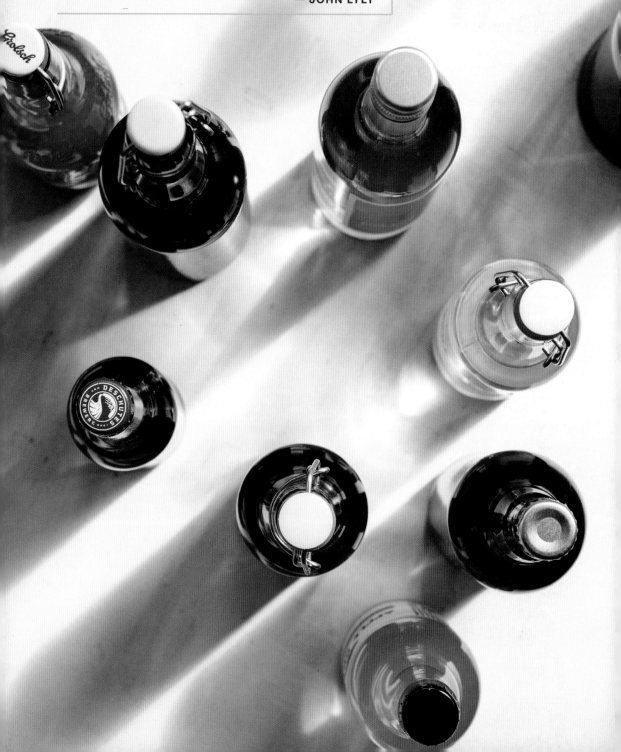

"As the best wine doth make the sharpest vinegar, so the deepest love turneth to the deadliest hate."

— JOHN LYLY

CHAPTER 3

ALCOHOL PRIMER
FOR THE
VINEGAR MAKER

F YOU ARE ALREADY A BREWER or a maker of other libations, then you have a treasure trove of opportunity to take that saison beer or homemade wine and make magic. If you aren't yet, then this is the beginning of your journey to becoming an acid alchemist. As you now understand, vinegar is a two-step fermentation, and the world's best vinegars start out with good ingredients, fermented into respectable wine, sake, cider, or other alcohol. You can start with ready-made alcohol; there are several recipes in this book that do so. However, to create the tastiest vinegars possible, you'll need to become a maker of alcohol. In this book, you'll be able to make vinegar without diving too deeply into the yeasty-boozy ferments. But if vinegar grabs your fancy, which I am afraid it very much can, it's important you know a little about this first step.

ALCOHOL STARTS WITH YEAST

Yeast is the single-celled fungus that brings us things like bread, wine, cider, and beer. It is found readily on the blossoms and fruit of plants. On some fruit, such as strawberries or apples, it may not be apparent. On others—such as grapes, blueberries, plums, prickly pears, and juniper berries—the white, powdery bloom you see on the skin is loaded with yeast.

Nectar has also been found to contain yeast; there are up to 400 million cells of yeast in less than an eighth of a teaspoon of nectar. Yeast isn't the only microbe present; our vinegar maker acetic acid bacteria is also there, waiting in the wings. The nectar in flower blossoms attracts pollinators like bumblebees, and the number of bee visits are believed to be a strong factor in the variety and concentration of yeasts found in and on fruit.

You have a couple of choices when it comes to making sure that your sugary liquid has a good yeast population to get it on its way: Either capture wild yeasts or use a commercial strain.

Capturing Wild Yeasts

Your first option is to simply leave fresh, unpasteurized juice in an open vessel and let the yeast that populate it, along with any that drop in, do the work. In most cases, the fruit you're using came with plenty of yeast ready to go to work, as long as you're not starting with pasteurized juice. Technically, wild yeasts from the air will make their way into any sugary juice, but it can be hit or miss. If you'd like to work with wild yeasts but have no access to raw juice, you can begin your vinegar project by making a wild yeast starter (see page 53). Making a starter also gives you a chance to "test" the yeasts you've

captured; they may be active and delicious or they may be faulty.

I often make these starters with blossoms. Flowers are full of nectar, which has sugar—and where there's sugar, there's yeast. I used to joke about all the little bee bottoms moving yeast around as they visited flowers; as it turns out, the yeasts in the nectar can actually enhance the flowers signal to the pollinators to attract them. One study found that bees spent significantly more time and energy on the flower with yeast than on the sterile (yeast-free) control flowers.[6] Another study found the yeasts themselves may rely on overwintering pollinators to complete their life cycle.[7]

To be a part of this wild yeast dance, you can make your own wild vinegar starters. A starter is a mini fermentation that gives you a preview of how well your wild yeasts will work on your batch of vinegar. You want to make sure it is a good starter before you use it. If it's quite active, you'll know that the yeasts are viable. You'll also have a chance to taste it. If it is boozy, that's a good sign. If it's sour and lactic, that means you caught lactic acid bacteria, which turns those sugars into lactic acid (not vinegar acid) rather than alcohol, and you don't want to use it.

I usually prefer spontaneous fermentation when I'm working with raw, fresh ingredients. However, in many of the recipes in this book, I add a yeast starter. I give you the option to choose a commercial yeast or a wild yeast starter. It's especially important to add a starter if you're working with a simultaneous ferment (page 81), because you want to make sure the alcohol gets off to a good start. Adding a starter is called pitching, which just means inoculating with a yeast (wild starter or commercial). Adding yeast is also necessary when you're using pasteurized

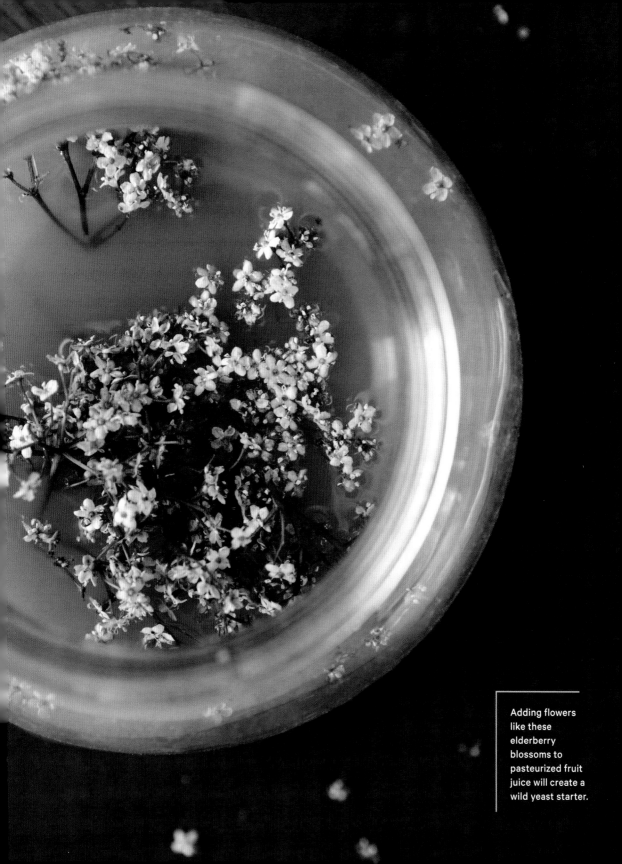

Adding flowers like these elderberry blossoms to pasteurized fruit juice will create a wild yeast starter.

juices or other liquids like corncob or corn husk brine (see page 184). In many old recipes, you will see baking yeast recommended, but I prefer brewing strains. Both are strains of *Saccharomyces cerevisiae*, as are many of the wild team. Team Wild often begins with the *Kloeckera apiculata* strains, which move in first and grow rapidly. They don't last long, though; they die out after the ethanol reaches about 2 percent. That's when the *Saccharomyces* strains take over. Other wild players might include *Torulopsis stella*, *Saccharomycodes ludwigii*, and *Candida* species.

Choosing a Commercial Yeast

For the purposes of vinegar making, you don't need a specific yeast. Basic wine or beer yeast, or even breadmaking yeast strains, all convert sugar to ethanol. They are generally strains of *Saccharomyces cerevisiae*. *Saccharo* means "to come from sugar," while *myces* means "from fungus." Finally, *cerevisiae* means "brewery." Now you see why it is often referred to as brewer's yeast or baker's yeast.

Nearly all of these yeast strains are bred for, among other things, alcohol tolerance that exceeds what you are targeting for vinegar. So you won't need to worry about picking a yeast strain that will poop out partway through the sugar-to-alcohol party. Nearly anything you can pick up at a local brewing shop will work, though some yeasts are easier to work with than others. Sparkling wine yeast is perhaps the easiest to find and one of the best to use for making vinegar. The name on the package will depend on the manufacturer. For example, Lalvin's version is called EC-1118 while Red Star's version is called Premier Cuvée. Both are the same Prise de Mousse strain. If those aren't available to you, look for any white wine yeast.

In the Red Star line, that could be either Côtes des Blanc or Premier Blanc or QA23 or ICV-D47 from Lalvin.

Unsure Which to Choose? Experiment!

Fermenters can be very opinionated about their yeast source. Some like the excitement and unpredictability of wild yeasts, while others feel that all yeasts were once wild, so why not use a predictable strain. I tend to walk on the wild side, but honestly, I don't limit myself to one camp. I use what I think will work best for the type of vinegar I am trying to achieve. Because so much of what I do is about discovery, I see failures as part of the territory.

That said, sometimes you don't want to mess around. Ingredients can be precious, because they are either limited or expensive. In such cases, you might be more comfortable using either a cultivated commercial yeast or a proven yeast—this can be a strain that you've caught in a starter jar and know works. I've heard working with wild yeasts described as trying to get a job done with volunteers. Wild yeasts can be exciting because the results are unknown. One concern people have when making alcohol with wild yeasts, though, is that some strains die off in the alcohol at a low ABV before all the sugar is eaten, or before the alcohol level is high enough to give you a strong enough percent acid.

I like to share recipes that I've had a number of successes with, but I also want this to be your adventure. You do you! If you love wild style, just substitute a wild yeast starter where I suggest a commercial yeast, or allow nature to take its course. By the same token, if I suggest wild yeast, feel free to pitch your favorite strain from the homebrew store.

FEEDING YEAST

Yeasts need food, which is mostly in the form of sugar. Since simple sugars start out trapped in fruits or grains, our first step is to free the sugars so that they are more accessible for the yeasts to consume. In the case of fruit, this means juicing or mashing them. If you're using fruit with a low sugar content, you should mash it to release its inherent sugar *and* add some sugar to achieve the right alcohol level. If you're upcycling leftover pomace from juicing, you can steep it in hot water for a few days to extract the sugar that's left, and also add a little sugar. But in all of these fruity situations, the simple sugar is there and ready to go to work.

In the case of grains, there is an additional step, because the sugars in grains aren't readily available to the yeasts. To free those sugars, we need the help of enzymes. These can be enlisted through the process of malting, as we see in beer making, or with the help of another microbe, a fungus called koji. See page 277 for details on the koji process.

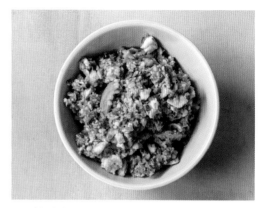

Add a little sugar to apple pomace before using it to make vinegar.

Another way to feed yeast is to use concentrates—syrups that are usually the result of removing water from an extract of the base material through boiling, distilling, or other means of evaporation. Date, rice, and maple syrups are examples, as is molasses. If you try to sprinkle yeast in these thick syrups, the yeast won't thrive because the syrups are too thick and have too much sugar. They need to be diluted with unchlorinated water (see page 54).

WILDCRAFTING BLOSSOM YEAST

As foraging or wildcrafting has become more popular, the concern is whether it is sustainable. The beautiful thing about yeast harvesting is you need very little of the plant material to get things going. Instead of uprooting entire plants, you pick a blossom or two. One small cluster of milkweed flowers, for example, will give you enough yeast and essence for a couple of quarts of vinegar. For more foraging tips, see Foraging for Flavor on page 232. Here are a few notes to start.

- Don't harvest blossoms from areas that have been sprayed with pesticides or herbicides.
- Remember that not every flower (or plant) is edible. Be sure to identify the plant and flower and use only the edible parts.
- Use flowers sparingly—especially at first—as some may cause digestive upset in some people.

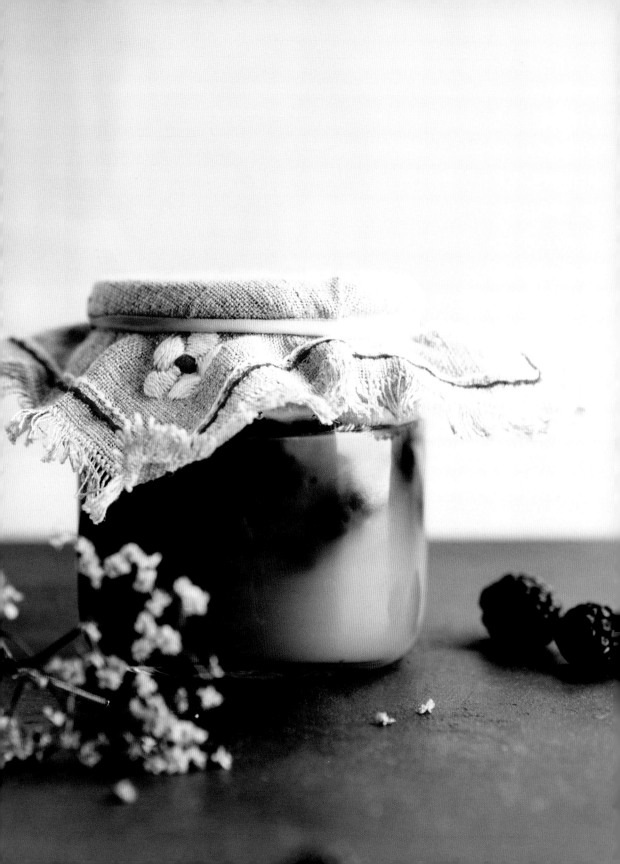

Making a Wild Yeast Starter

In our book *The Big Book of Cidermaking*, my husband, Christopher, and I give you in-depth information on foraging for wild yeast. I use a lot of botanical and blossom yeasts to ferment regular grocery store apple juice into cider and then vinegar. This is taking the idea of DIY herbal vinegars to another level, as it is the herbs and botanicals that are part of creating the vinegar. For example, two floral vinegars that we enjoy are lilac vinegar and dandelion blossom vinegar. See the Lilac Vinegar recipe on page 122 to harness flower power for wild floral vinegars.

You will need a pint jar, its lid, and pasteurized fruit juice—generally I use apple or grape. The juice ensures that the yeast have enough nutrients to get off to a good start. (If using your own homemade juices, you will need to pasteurize them first.)

1. Sterilize a clean 1-pint jar and its lid (or another container that has a tight-fitting lid or is capable of holding an airlock) by submerging it in boiling water for 10 minutes.

2. Using tongs, transfer the hot jar to a clean towel, placing it right-side up. Allow the jar to cool before filling, to avoid breaking it.

3. Using pasteurized juice from a bottle that has just been opened, fill the jar three-quarters full with juice. For a pint jar, this will be 1½ cups (355 mL) apple juice.

4. Add fresh botanicals, berries, or flower petals to the juice in the jar. We use about ⅓ cup (71 g) fruit for 1½ cups (355 mL) juice. For flower petals, we've found that 5 to 20 grams is often sufficient. This can be around ¼ cup to 1 cup of petals. As little as 1 to 2 grams work (which can be just a few sunflower petals), but if you want a stronger flavor, use more.

5. Cover the jar with a lid and tighten. The carbon dioxide produced by the fermentation process will need to escape, so the jar will need to be burped once or twice a day.

6. Let it sit at room temperature or cooler; wild yeast do better in cool, slow fermentations. Stir or shake the mixture three times a day. You may begin to notice bubbling in 2 to 3 days, though it could take 2 weeks or more in cool temperatures. As the yeast populations grow, the bubbling will become more active, and you'll be able to smell and even taste the solution to see what kind of flavors are developing. If it's pleasing, you can pour this into the base juice/liquid that you'll be making vinegar with. If you don't see any activity after the second week, the wild yeast may not be strong. You can continue to wait; it may still take. If you begin to see mold growth or a layer of surface yeast growing on top (see Troubleshooting, page 274), you will need to toss the starter, sterilize the jar, and begin again.

7. When it's done fermenting, store with a tightened lid in the refrigerator. Bring the starter and your base liquid to room temperature before inoculating, to prevent yeast shock (which will kill some of it). When ready to use, shake the starter to mix in lees, then pour it through a strainer to filter out starter materials. If you choose a wild yeast starter for a recipe, you'll see the recipes call for ½ cup starter. If you don't intend to use it for anything else, go ahead and use the whole amount; otherwise store in a small airtight jar, with as little airspace as possible, in the refrigerator. Under anaerobic conditions, starter will last at least a year, and often longer. (When using starter that is more than a year old, double the amount.)

VINEGAR WON'T SOLVE YOUR ALCOHOL PROBLEM

The alcohol you make for vinegar doesn't have to be most delicious libation ever. Nevertheless, making vinegar shouldn't be seen as a way to make use of an undrinkable batch of homemade wine, beer, or cider. Generally, it cannot fix something that is broken. With alcohol, you need to understand there are two types of bad. One is it is not tasty, but the faults are minor. The other kind is more of the off, rank, contaminated nature. This can be caused by anything from bacteria to mold in your batch—toss those brews.

Now that I've told you the rule, I am going to say I break it all the time. For years, Christopher and I have been surprised at how some of our not-the-most-delicious cider has been transformed into oh-so-delicious vinegars. We made two early-summer wild blossom ciders—a rose-valerian cider and a blackberry blossom–wild oat cider—that weren't so drinkable. I mixed them in a two-gallon jar, tossed in an MOV, then set it on a shelf and forgot about it. I figured, I have to try; worst-case scenario, it just gets dumped.

Four months later, it had taken on flavors from the flowers. It was interesting, complex, one of the most delicious vinegars we've ever made, and completely not repeatable—an enchanting example of the zen of fermentation.

Measuring and Adjusting Sugar Content

To produce the vinegar you want, you'll need to be able to measure the sugar content of your base ingredients. The original sugar content of the juice determines its ultimate alcohol level, and the alcohol level determines the final acidity level of the vinegar. Being able to adjust the amount of sugar in the base ingredients will enable you to produce alcohol that is in the right range of ABV.

As we learned in Chapter 2, the final ABV should be between 5 and 9 percent. A low-ABV alcohol will result in a vinegar that is not stable and is susceptible to unwanted microbes, like *E. coli* or botulism. Conversely, an ABV above 9 percent is too high for acetic bacteria to thrive.

ADDING SUGAR TO INCREASE THE ATTAINABLE ABV. If your starting juice has a very low sugar content, you will want to supplement with some sugar (page 59) or reduce the water content by boiling it down or by freezing and pouring off the water. For example, raspberries, elderberries, and fruit or vegetable scraps have little sugar to ferment, so their attainable alcohol level is only around 2 to 3 percent. This gives you a very weak vinegar that could spoil; bringing up the sugar level will yield a better final product.

ADDING WATER TO DECREASE SUGAR LEVEL. Base ingredients with high levels of sugar might need to be diluted. Concentrated sugars such as boiled cider syrup, molasses, honey, and other thick syrups are examples of this. Even microbes have their limits; this is why old-school fruit preserves relied on sugar.

Knowing how much water to add can be figured out pretty simply by measuring the specific gravity with a hydrometer (see page 58). You'll need to dilute, test, and likely repeat until you have a ratio that you can apply to the batch you are making. The good news is I've already measured the specific gravity for all the recipes in this book. If you have a syrup that doesn't have a recipe in this book, follow the instructions on page 58 to determine the specific gravity of the syrup you'd like to work with.

SPECIFIC GRAVITY, BRIX, AND PREDICTING THE FUTURE?

There are two ways to measure the sugars present in juice and fermenting alcohol: Brix and specific gravity. Which method you choose depends on what kind of process you're comfortable with. Some of us just like knowing and using this kind of information to better control the process, while others simply rely on their senses. For thousands of years, people have been making vinegar by instinct, and we can, too. Taste each stage. Take note of the sweetness and then the alcohol and acids that develop. As you do so, you'll train your palate to recognize sugary base materials that are too thin to make a solid vinegar. Taking measurements can help you train your palate.

Brix

The Brix scale measures how much the sugar in the liquid refracts light; the Brix number is obtained by dropping juice on the prism of a handheld refractometer. The Brix number is then used to calculate the amount of alcohol

> For thousands of years, people have been making vinegar by instinct, and we can, too.

the liquid is capable of producing. In general, a happy place for vinegar is 12.4 to 20.0 degrees Brix (see page 56 for more details).

Although it's a handy tool, you should know there are a couple of challenges with using a Brix refractometer for making vinegar. Once fermentation begins and any ethanol is present, Brix refractometers don't work anymore. It is also important to know that it's calibrated against pure sucrose, so it can have trouble reading cloudy liquids like apple juice. This can be worked around by filtering the juice; see page 102. I never used a refractometer when I was working with pure fruit juices, but when I started working with vegetables and some scrap recipes that produced base liquids that were too thick for a hydrometer, I found that filtering a few drops from the base made it possible to get a sugar measurement.

You should be aware that there are separate alcohol-specific refractometers—because alcohol and sugar have a different refractive index. I have never used one but can see where it would be useful. If you look for one that is alcohol specific, make sure that it measures *actual alcohol content*. Product descriptions can be confusing; some say they measure alcohol when they are actually measuring sugar (and therefore are just predictive of the potential alcohol content).

Measuring Brix with a Refractometer

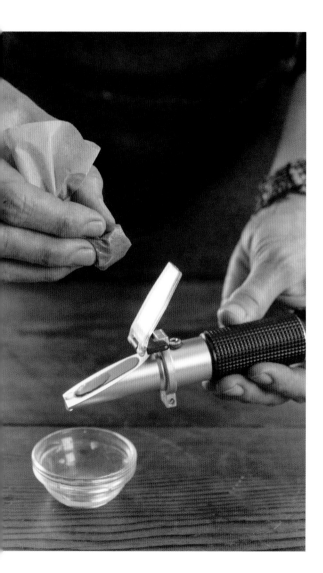

Use a refractometer to measure Brix, as expressed by degrees. On the Brix scale, 1 degree Brix (1°Bx) is 1 gram of sucrose per 100 grams of liquid.

1. Make sure the water and the sample (juice) are at room temperature.

2. Calibrate the refractometer with pure clean water before reading the sample. To do this, place the drops on the view plate and close the lid so the water spreads. Point toward bright light and adjust the focus of the eyepiece to zero.

3. Open the plate and wipe it with a soft, dry, dust-free cloth (like an eyeglass cleaning cloth).

4. Use a 50/50 mixture of water and juice. Mix well, then pour a bit into a clean coffee filter. Squeeze a drop or two onto the cleaned view plate.

5. Close the lid and let the liquid spread to cover the view plate. Hold the refractometer up to a bright light source and take note of where the color line shows distinctly.

There are tables and conversion charts online, but for vinegar making I try to keep the Brix between 12.4 and 20.0 degrees. This translates to a specific gravity of 1.050 to 1.080, which puts you right in the ballpark of 5 to 9 percent alcohol by volume (ABV)—your vinegar-making sweet spot. My happy place is 17 degrees Brix.

Specific Gravity

Specific gravity (SG) describes the relative density of the juice, compared to water. Why do you want to know the density of your juice? Because as the juice ferments, the sugars are converted to ethanol and carbon dioxide in roughly equal amounts, lowering the density of the juice. By measuring the specific gravity during the fermentation stage, you can get a pretty good idea of how much of the sugar has been devoured by the yeasts and converted to alcohol (or alcohol and vinegar, if you're doing a simultaneous-type ferment). This measurement is made with a hydrometer; using either a chart or the marks on the side of the hydrometer, it's easy to translate a SG to the amount of sugar something contains, which then tells you how much alcohol it will finally have when the fermentation is complete.

Water has a SG of 1.000, so any sugar present raises that level. Apple, pear, and other juices have specific gravities that usually range from 1.045 to 1.065. This gives you the (expected) ABV, which is a guide to the future acidity. For example, if the hydrometer predicts a 6 percent ABV, this is the alcohol level the juice is capable of producing, and an indicator that the vinegar has the potential to be 6 percent acid (more likely, it will be closer to 5 percent, because the oxygen in the process can cause some of the alcohol to evaporate before it becomes acid). I use SG measurements when I'm making vinegar; it's an easy step and it helps inform my choices when I'm making unusual or scrap vinegars. As when you're brewing beer or making cider or wine, there is a certain amount of wiggle room, but these measurements help us know what sugar ballpark we are in, without needing to send off samples at any stage of the making—from juice to alcohol to the final vinegar—to labs for exact (and expensive) testing. Luckily, simple and inexpensive hydrometers work well and measure both alcohol and sugar content. And if you are curious, there are tables online to convert degrees Brix to specific gravity (see the link on page 285).

Keep in mind that you can't go back and get the specific gravity or Brix measurement once the fermentation is under way. To know that exactly, you would need the help of a lab, although you can buy photometric kits that promise to help you do this at home. For the purposes of artisan vinegar, a close approximation will get you well within the ranges. If you're starting with finished wine, cider, beer, or other brews, you won't need to go through this process.

TIPS FOR USING A HYDROMETER

Another thing to know is that hydrometers are often calibrated to solutions at 60°F/15°C. Unless your liquid is around that temperature, your measurement will be off a bit. Second, the gas bubbles will attach to the bottom and sides of the hydrometer, giving it a boost upward and artificially raising the SG level reading. Shake or swirl the hydrometer in the liquid to dislodge the bubbles from the bottom and sides. This also helps knock down the bubbles on the surface of the liquid, to provide a more accurate reading. If you have adjusted for these things and are still getting a reading below 1.045, you need a sugar source to bump up your reading.

Measuring Specific Gravity

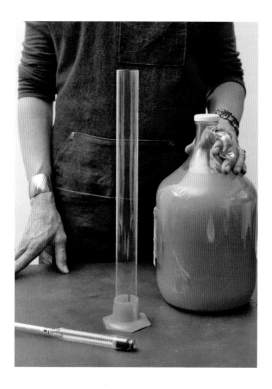

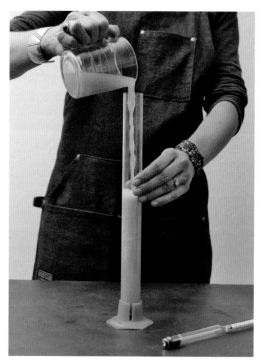

1. Assemble your equipment. You will need a wine thief to extract the base liquid for testing, a hydrometer jar, and a hydrometer.

2. Fill the hydrometer jar halfway. Carefully place the hydrometer in the jar, then add enough liquid to sufficiently float the hydrometer.

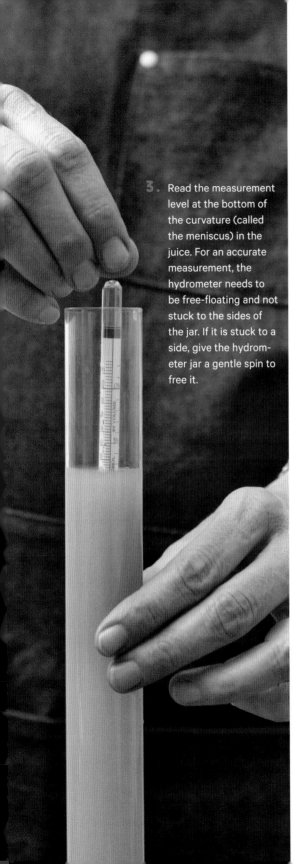

3. Read the measurement level at the bottom of the curvature (called the meniscus) in the juice. For an accurate measurement, the hydrometer needs to be free-floating and not stuck to the sides of the jar. If it is stuck to a side, give the hydrometer jar a gentle spin to free it.

Adjusting the Specific Gravity

TOO LOW. When the specific gravity of your juice is less than 1.045, the minimum needed to produce a high enough ABV to preserve the resulting vinegar naturally, you will want to make adjustments. This process is called chaptalization (or, sometimes, enrichment). In vinegar making, it is done before fermentation. It can also be done in stages, throughout the fermentation, so as not to overwhelm the yeast with too much sugar at once. Depending on your base, you may need to add sugar in your raw juice or other base liquid to bring it to the target SG level. To produce a 5 percent alcohol, the SG should be 1.038. For me, this is the minimum reading; I like to have a little wiggle room, given a very small amount of the alcohol produced becomes the residual alcohol needed for a long-lasting vinegar. For stable vinegars, I shoot for an SG measurement of 1.040 to 1.055.

TOO HIGH. This is much less likely, but what if the specific gravity of your juice is too high? If your SG is above 1.085 (predicting a level above 9 percent), you can either water down your juice or stop the fermentation before it reaches full dryness by adding the vinegar mother before the alcohol is fully fermented.

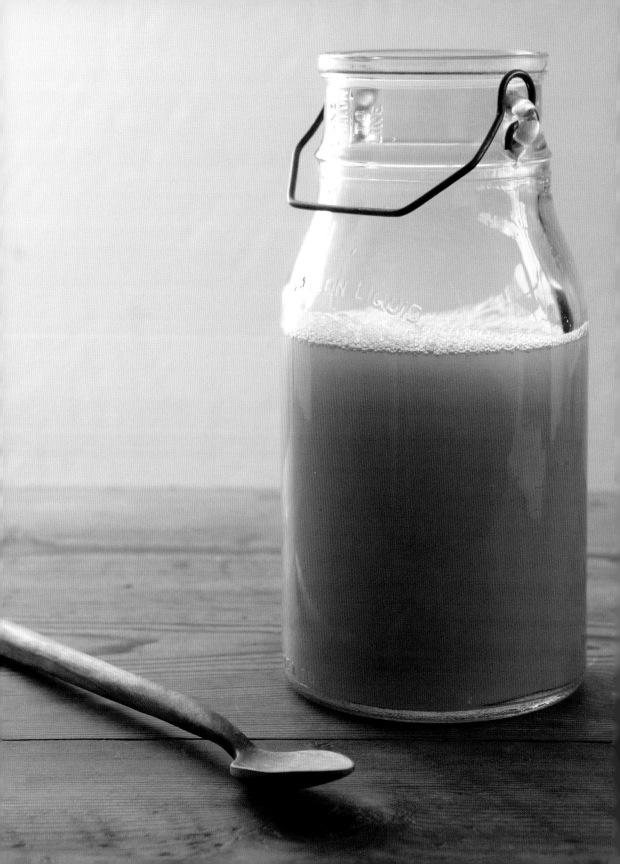

How to Raise the SG of Juice by Adding Sugar

Adding sugar is probably the simplest way to raise the specific gravity. The math is based on readily available white sugar (or its less-refined equivalent), but any basic sugar will work.

1. Separate out 1 quart (946 mL) of juice.

2. Add some of the juice to a hydrometer jar and float the hydrometer to take a reading. Note both the specific gravity reading and the likely ABV when finished.

3. It's time to do some math! For about a 1 percent increase in ABV, you should add 23 grams of sugar to every quart of juice. So, for example, if our SG reading was 1.038 (5 percent ABV) and we want to raise that to 6 percent ABV, we need to raise the SG to 1.046. That works out to about 6 teaspoons (23 g) of sugar per quart (946 mL) of base juice/liquid.

4. Pour the juice back into the quart jar, add the amount of sugar you calculated for your situation, and stir to combine.

5. Add some of the sugared juice to a narrow, clear container and float the hydrometer in it.

6. Note the rise in specific gravity to make sure it has risen to the target level. If not, make adjustments.

How to Raise the SG of Juice by Boiling It Down

The good thing with this method is that you're not adding any outside sugar source, so you're keeping the flavors unadulterated. This is great if you have plenty of fruit you're turning into vinegar. Determining how long it will take to reduce the water content to a level you want is a less-than-exact calculation, but this is the basic process.

1. Put the fruit juice in a pot and bring to a simmer over medium-high heat without a lid. Note the starting level of the juice.

2. Reduce the heat to keep the juice at a low simmer, and keep the lid off.

3. Stir the juice now and then as the water steams off, and watch the starting juice level to gauge how much it has reduced. I find that reducing it by one-fifth to one-quarter of its original volume is good. Once you get below that, you're starting to get into thicker syrups and concentrates. Cool it to 60°F/15°C and take another SG reading.

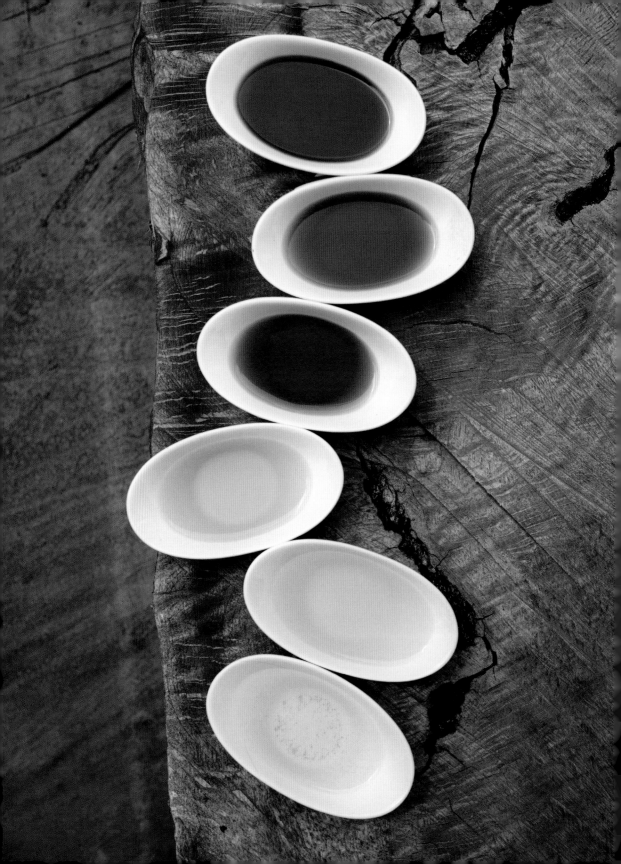

CHAPTER 4

LET'S MAKE
VINEGAR

E'RE ALMOST THERE. This chapter will introduce you to the tools and equipment you'll need to make vinegar and control the process. You'll also get a step-by-step tour of all the methods you'll come across in the recipes. A good understanding of the methods will free you to create your own unique flavors. Finally, this chapter will explain aging and bottling. From this point on, you will be ready to begin your own personal acid trip.

START WITH QUALITY INGREDIENTS

All it really takes to make vinegar is a base substrate (essentially, any ingredient with sugar in it), some water, and some microbes. You can make vinegar from any number of ingredients: fruit, flowers, grains, honey, sap, vegetables . . . the list goes on and on. Whatever ingredients you use should be as fresh and free from chemicals as possible. (Don't use juices with preservatives for example.) High-quality inputs work magic all the way through the process.

When the recipes call for water, I specify unchlorinated water. Check to see whether your town's water treatment facility uses plain chlorine—which can be boiled, or dissipated out, by leaving an open jug of water out overnight—or chloramine, which will not dissipate and must be filtered. Don't use distilled water; fermentation needs the trace amounts of calcium. For those of you with hard water, look at that—it's good for something after all!

The two types of microbes at work in vinegar making are yeast and acetic bacteria, both of which are pervasive in our environment. To ensure a better chance of success, though, I suggest you add a little yeast and a little acetic bacteria to get things off to a good start. Each recipe gives you the option of using either a commercial yeast or a wild yeast starter. (There's no judgment here—it's your adventure, so choose the method you prefer.) Each recipe also calls for some type of starter. Feel free to use a previous mother, unpasteurized vinegar from the store, or vinegar from another batch you've made. And should you want to play around with using nothing, I give you permission to do that, as well. I find the best way to learn is to push at all the boundaries and see what works for you.

EQUIPMENT FOR MAKING VINEGAR AT HOME

What will you need? Not much; mostly patience and a vessel. A vessel with a wide-open top is not only better for the required oxygen but also makes moving the mother and cleaning the vessel easier. For example, a gallon jar is better than a gallon bottle. If you do use a bottle, don't fill it to the neck. Instead, fill it to the widest part—vinegar making is all about exposing as much surface area to oxygen as possible. This goes against everything you've been told about

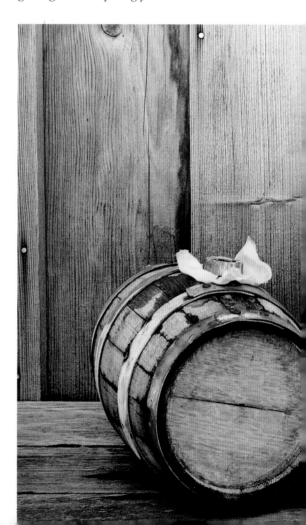

> "Unless the vessel be pure, everything which is poured into it will turn sour." —HORACE

how to properly ferment alcohol or lactic acid vegetables. Let's look at some container options and the materials they are made of.

Jars, Barrels, and Ceramic Vessels

GLASS JARS are easy to use, easy to procure, and easy to clean. The best part is that you can see what's going on with your ferment. Most of the vinegar I make is in glass jars with wide openings.

WOODEN BARRELS are classic vinegar fermentation vessels. You can find barrels with a spigot in the bottom and a wide hole in the top, just for this purpose; I use these for our continuous brews. (See Resources, page 285.) Regular closed barrels (no oxygen) are also used in aging. I love the subtle flavor that wood imparts.

There are a few things to understand about working with wood. The first is that it becomes

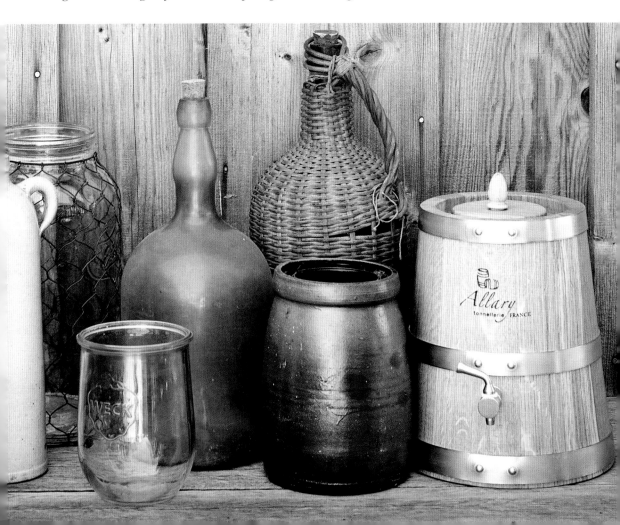

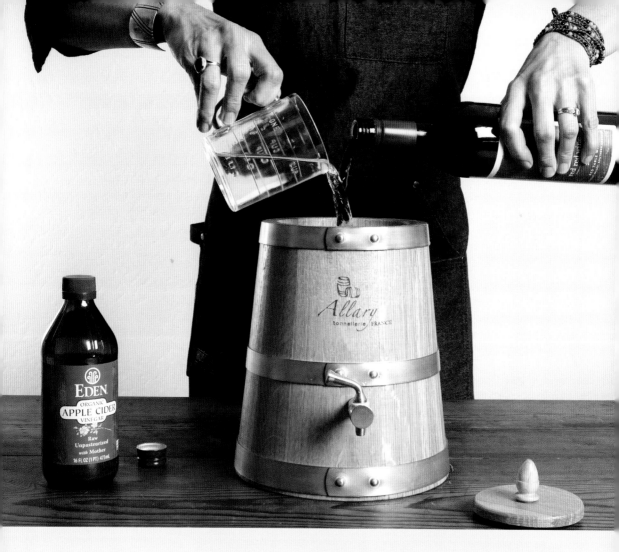

CONTINUOUS VINEGAR BREWING

A continuous-brew vinegar pot has many advantages. Probably the best is that any unfinished alcoholic beverage at the bottom of a can or bottle can be upcycled into vinegar: Instead of getting poured down the drain, the leftovers go into the pot. Whenever you need a little vinegar, you simply open the spigot. You'll want to stick to like alcohol, though: If you're a wine drinker, you'll never need to buy wine vinegar again. Beer drinkers may discover a love for malty or hoppy beer vinegar. This is also a way to make vinegar from higher-proof alcohols like sake, wine, or spirits that would otherwise need diluting.

The first vinegar production in France, called the Orleans method, was a form of continuous brewing. To do something similar, use a barrel or vinegar pot with a spigot on the bottom to brew your first batch of vinegar. Once it's finished, you generally remove about 25 percent of the vinegar from the spigot. You can do this every few weeks. And like the vinegar makers in Orleans, you'll need to remove the mother every so often, lest she fill the whole space. See Setting up a Continuous-Brew Vinegar Pot (page 90) for complete instructions, and refer to the kitchen-counter Boerhaave method (page 94) for more continuous-brew ideas.

very much a part of the "live" fermentation, as microbes take up residence in the porous wood. This is to your advantage when it's a community of bacteria and yeasts that you desire for good vinegar. Fermentation educator Nicole Easterday shared that she'd kept her wood barrel stored with just water in it for a while. It was so well inoculated that when she was ready to use it and put wine in the barrel, it began producing a cellulose mother and vinegar immediately with no additional starter. This can work both ways, though; wood can be a challenge, should undesirable microbes move in.

Barrels are great for continuous brewing, because they need to stay saturated in order to be watertight. A barrel should never be left empty; it should always be kept three-quarters full, at the very least, of liquid. My husband, Christopher, and I learned this the hard way. Under storage conditions, the barrels dry out, the staves shrink, and the barrels leak. If you'll be storing it, be sure to fill it with a solution of 4 grams of citric acid or 8 grams of potassium metabisulfite per gallon of water. Fill it completely, and it top off as needed during storage; this will keep your barrel from leaking. The downside is that over the long haul, this solution will slowly leach the oak flavor from the wood. (Dried barrels sometimes can be salvaged by a good long soak, with varying results.)

CERAMIC VESSELS are not only functional but beautiful. Ceramic vinegar pots (with a bottom spigot) are also time-honored vessels for the vinegar maker. Some glazes are as impermeable as glass, but other traditional types of vessels "breathe" (just not in the same way as wood does). We have long been advocates of fermenting in traditional ceramic vessels for this very reason. These old-school vessels not only work well but also infuse their own character into the ferment. These can be used for single batches but are also great to keep on the counter for a continuous vinegar.

Considering Materials

If using plastic, be sure to use HDPE food-grade containers, as some plastics can corrode when exposed to vinegar. For example, polycarbonates will corrode, and they contain the controversial chemical BPA. The food-grade rule goes both for making and storage.

Containers made of high-quality stainless steel are good. There are more than 100 grades of stainless steel, as determined by its strength and resistance to corrosion and oxidation. Stainless steel fermenters are usually a 304 or 316 grade, which is what you want in fermentation; lower grades, which are common in cookware, won't stand up to the acid. So don't assume your stockpot will work, unless you know the grade. All other metals are easily corroded by vinegar—bad for both the vessel and the vinegar—causing not only off flavors but, in some cases, toxins. The brewing industry uses stainless steel vessels in all shapes and sizes. If you look into kombucha brewing, you will find countertop vessels that can be used for continuous-brew vinegar pots.

SPIGOTS. For a continuous-brew setup, you'll want a vessel with a spigot at the bottom. Just be sure that spigot is of good quality. Remember this is vinegar, which is highly acidic. The spigot should be made of corrosion-resistant material, such as stainless steel or wood, and free of all paints or epoxies.

Keep It Covered

To cover your vessel, you'll want something that is permeable by air but not fruit flies. You can use cloth—just be sure the weave is tight enough to not allow fruit flies. A clean cotton flour sack dish towel works, as does a square of muslin. I found that basket-style coffee filters can be invaluable for topping jars; they meet all the above criteria. They're also good to have on hand for filtering the vinegar (see page 102 for more on this). I use large rubber bands, cotton string, or a threaded metal jar band (for mason jars) to keep the coverings tight and in place. Make sure your rubber band or string fits snugly, so that fruit flies can't squeeze through. I often use two rubber bands, one on the threaded area of the jar and the other just under it. When using string, I wrap it a few times before tying it—again to make it harder for a fruit fly to sneak in.

Tools for Measuring pH and Sugar Content

The following measurement devices will step up the control you have in the process, but great vinegar can be made without them. Decisions about which tools to invest in are completely personal and have to do with how you like to work.

Measuring pH tells you the acidity or alkalinity of your vinegar. I use this measurement twice in vinegar making. First, I like to know the pH of the base I'm starting with, whether that's unfermented juice or alcohol, so that I can monitor the progress of the brew. If the pH starts above 5.0 or 6.0, I add acid—be it from lemon juice or the raw vinegar starter—early

in the vinegar fermentation process. A low pH helps keep the brew from getting an overgrowth of kahm yeast, mold, or other spoilers that come with the open air, during the alcohol, or vinegar, fermentation. A high pH will make your brew more susceptible to surface yeast.

Measuring sugar content is a great indicator of what the final acid percentage your vinegar will have, which you can read all about on page 39.

PH INDICATOR STRIPS are an inexpensive and easy way to check pH. Simply dip the strip in the liquid and compare the resulting color to a color grid. Get strips that are for brewing or cheese making, as they will have smaller incremental measurements of the pH range. You will know, for example, if your batch is around 4.6 instead of trying to fathom if it is pH 4.0 or 5.0. These strips are not considered highly accurate but work well for all my fermentation purposes.

A PH METER is a handheld meter that is calibrated against a known solution. The probe is then dipped into the vinegar solution, and the reading is shown on a screen. They are a fun gadget but can be expensive.

A HYDROMETER measures the specific gravity of a liquid, which is how much sugar it contains. The hydrometer is a weighted glass tool that looks like a bloated thermometer and is made to float in a liquid. It has two parts: a cylinder that you fill with your liquid and the glass hydrometer itself. The hydrometer is placed in the liquid, and how far the hydrometer sinks into the liquid shows how much sugar the liquid contains. For more about how to measure specific gravity, see page 58.

A REFRACTOMETER measures sucrose and gives you a Brix number. It is a fun tool but isn't strictly necessary. You can read about how and why you would use one on page 56. It gives you the same information as the hydrometer.

Additional Equipment

There are a few pieces of bonus equipment that, although not at all necessary, you may want in your home vinegar works.

A SPRAY BOTTLE filled with 80 proof clear alcohol, like vodka or gin. This can be invaluable for quick sanitizing as you are working. A few spritzes on top of a vinegar in progress can also help control surface yeast or mold growth. (See Troubleshooting, page 274.)

A RACKING CANE with a bit of tubing, or just a bit of tubing, is invaluable in siphoning vinegar off the sediment if you are looking to bottle clear vinegar.

A JUICER comes in handy. You can make all the recipes in this book without a juicer by procuring fresh-pressed apple cider (for apple cider vinegar) or making mashes with the various fruits and vegetables. However, with a juicer you can make and ferment juice from any fruit or vegetable that comes your way.

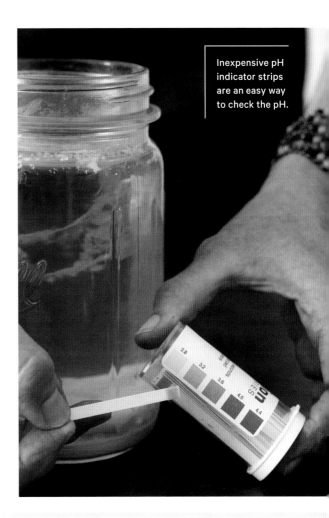

Inexpensive pH indicator strips are an easy way to check the pH.

WAITER, THERE'S A (FRUIT) FLY IN MY VINEGAR!

Don't worry: It won't drink too much. Seriously, although a full-on infestation could be a problem, it's not a huge issue to find a few fruit flies in your vinegar. They're really just more of an annoyance than a problem. Here in southern Oregon, late summer through midwinter is our fruit fly season. Unsurprisingly, that coincides with our brewing season. I watch the vinegar containers diligently during this time of year, because sometimes I need to take extra measures to ensure the fruit flies stay out of the ferment. This might include taping down the edges of the cloth or filter paper. If you're using a mason jar, tightening a metal jar band over the cloth or filter or paper is most effective.

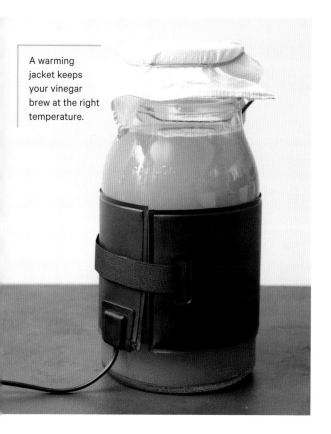

A warming jacket keeps your vinegar brew at the right temperature.

THERMOMETERS. Because vinegar's ideal spot is just slightly higher than room temperature, it's helpful to know what temperature you're working with. This is especially important if you find you're having issues with surface yeast (which is undesirable) or the slow growth of desirable yeast. A stick-on thermometer strip for each vessel is an inexpensive and helpful piece of equipment, even if it's not strictly necessary.

WARMING JACKET. Kombucha suppliers sell warming jackets to wrap on jars or vessels for brewing kombucha. If you're serious about making vinegar and your brewing environment is too cool, these can be a good tool.

FRUIT AND VEGETABLE STRAINER. A strainer (also known as a food mill) can be very handy for pressing out vinegar solids, especially in the cases of whole-fruit vinegars and amazake-based vinegars. Otherwise, use a fine-mesh sieve or a colander and high thread count cheesecloth.

KEEP THINGS CLEAN

A clean start is key. Use only ingredients that are free of chemicals and preservatives, and clean equipment. Be sure to sanitize your equipment, especially if you're starting at the first stage of fermentation—juice (sugary liquid) to alcohol. Yeast ferments can get contaminated by spoilers that will ruin them. To reduce chances of introducing unwanted bacteria from your equipment, soak all tools for at least 2 minutes in a homemade sanitizing solution—I tablespoon chlorine bleach diluted in I gallon of water. An alternative is a no-rinse brewing sanitizer, like Star San; simply mix the sanitizer with water, dunk equipment into the solution, and allow it to air-dry. My favorite sanitizing tool is a spray bottle filled with 80 proof (40 percent alcohol) clear alcohol like vodka. (Higher alcohol content isn't better in this case; at higher proofs, the alcohol can evaporate before killing unwanted bacteria.) I spritz this on tools and allow it to air-dry.

Bonus tip: Use that alcohol spritz to control surface yeast. Spray a light mist on the surface and side walls any time you see a film of yeast, and it usually gives up. Stop spritzing when it is no longer a problem.

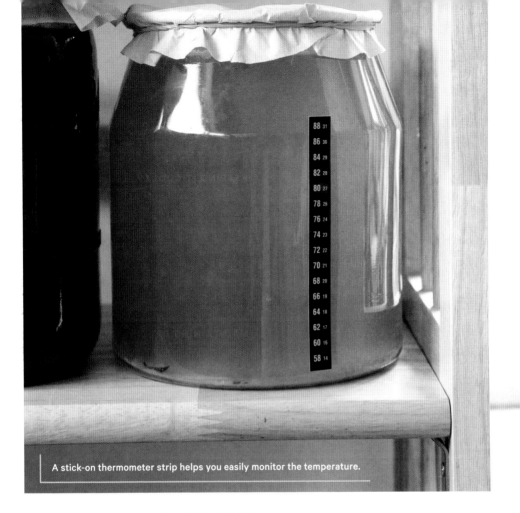

A stick-on thermometer strip helps you easily monitor the temperature.

A COZY, WARM SPOT, BUT NO SUNBATHING

Just like the bacteria involved in other types of fermentation, vinegar bacteria thrive in a particular environment. First of all, a bit of shade is best. The ambient light in your house won't hamper the fermentation, but vinegar bacteria are sensitive to ultraviolet light, so keep clear fermenting vessels out of direct sunlight. Aging vinegar should be kept someplace that's as dark as possible.

Getting the Temperature Right

More important is giving your acetobacters the proper temperature, right from the beginning. This will result in good acid production early in the ferment, which means you'll have fewer problems with surface yeasts and vinegar eels (see page 275).

WARM AND IDEAL. Technically, the acetobacters will survive and carry out fermentation across a large range of temperatures: from 43° to 95°F/6° to 35°C. However, they *prefer* a warm, cozy, environment—honestly, the kind of temperatures we also thrive in. Think of a lazy, late-summer day, 82°F/28°C. They actually like it a little warmer than we might keep our home: the optimal range is between 75° and 86°F/25° and 30°C, especially when the ferment is just getting started, with the ultimate sweet spot being 82°F/28°C.

COOL BUT RISKY. The low temperature range is 50° to 66°F/10° to 34°C—an acceptable range but one that puts you into that slower, higher-risk camp. The bottom range of 43° to 50°F/6° to 10°C is technically the minimum temperature needed for fermentation to take place and, in my experience, too cold to really get things going. I do, however, find this can be a good range for aging once your vinegar is bottled.

HOT AND DEADLY. It's important for the ferment to not get *too* warm. Growth becomes a problem for some of the bacteria at 95°F/35°C. At 101° to 105°F/38° to 41°C, most, if not all, bacteria will die, and any yeast still alive will become hyperactive. This can lead to significant flavor loss, as the esters leave with the significant amount of CO_2 being created. Finally, at about 113°F/45°C the yeasts die as well, and the mother will also die off if this temperature is sustained.

Ways to Regulate Temperature

The first simple trick is to get a thermometer strip that sticks to your vessel—like the kind that goes on an aquarium. This will give you an idea of the brew temperature. From there, you can see how the brew responds when it's placed in different locations around your home—the top of the fridge, on the water heater, or wherever you put it.

WARMING THE BREW. If your brew isn't reaching its ideal temperature, try a warming jacket (see page 70). Alternatively, you can put the vessel into an insulated cooler with a seed-starting mat or a heating pad that is controlled by an external thermostat. At the most

basic, you can place jars of hot water in the cooler once a day.

KEEPING IT COOL. Although you're more likely to have problems keeping your batch warm enough, extreme heat conditions may also pose a problem. If so, you'll want to find the coolest spot available for your vinegar vessel. This could be on a tile floor, under a bed, in a cooler with ice packs during the heat of the day, or even in the refrigerator for part of the day if things heat way up.

MAINTAINING PRECISE CONTROL. For the ultimate control, you can place the jar in a water bath with an aquarium heating element set to 82°F/28°C and an aquarium air pump to circulate the water. This will also work with an immersion circulator. If you do this, put 1 tablespoon of citric acid in every 3 gallons of water in the water bath to avoid algae growth.

The great thing about this method is that it can be used to keep the ferment at the proper temperature in any climate—including in warm climates, where the ferment should be kept cooler than the ambient air. To do that, set up the water bath in a picnic cooler to keep the hot air from further warming the water.

Working at a Larger Scale, with More Variety

The suggestions so far assume a small, movable batch. I simply have too many batches going in varying sizes to keep in my house's few warmer nooks and crannies. As a result, they mostly have to ferment in my fermentation space, which runs cooler than optimal most of the year. I'm still able to produce excellent vinegar, though, mostly because I always make sure

I'm starting each batch as warm as possible. I might set up a heater or a small heating pad, as needed, to give a new batch a head start. Once I see a mother, or have tasted that the new vinegar is acidic and I know it's well under way, I take the risk of fermenting at that cooler temperature. At this point, I'm not worried about spoilers moving in; once the microbes involved in fermenting have established a dominant population, it's very unlikely that unwanted bacteria will gain a foothold. I find the slower, cooler ferment during the second part of the fermentation also leads to deeper, mellow flavors. As in all fermentation, temperature is one of your main control points; it really depends on how much influence you want over the process and the final product.

WAYS TO MAKE VINEGAR

Ways to make vinegar range from the time-honored slow surface methods to pumping as much oxygen in as you can to speed things up. There are also several places to step into the vinegar-making process. You can start from the very beginning, with raw, whole produce, such as apples (maybe even pick them yourself). You can start with a quantity of kitchen scraps from your food preparations (you can save them up in the freezer, a bit at a time). You can skip that and still control both fermentation cycles by starting from juice, be it apple, coconut, or beet.

Or you can jump in at the acetic fermentation stage by simply procuring ready-made alcohol.

Surface Methods of Vinegar Making

Also called the slow method, surface ferments are just what they sound like. The surface of the ferment is exposed to oxygen. I say *methods* in the plural but really, they are variations on a theme. The bacteria, which require oxygen, do all the work at the surface of the liquid where they access the oxygen. Slowly over time, all the liquid is converted to vinegar. This is how humans have been making vinegar for a long time, and it works—it just *takes* a long time.

We might live in a culture of instant gratification, but I believe that anticipation can make the final product much more satisfying. It brings a sense of occasion every time you use your final product, having had the experience of tasting the flavors through the progression of the fermentation. Many people argue this slow, easy method (and its slow-acting microbes) makes a better-tasting vinegar. The liquid is also slowly evaporating as it turns from alcohol to vinegar, which helps to concentrate the flavors. As you'll learn on page 110, young vinegars are harsh, and the longer a vinegar is aged, the gentler it will become. I suspect part of what happens with this slower method is that there's already some of that mellowing taking place.

VINEGAR IS A TWO-STEP FERMENTATION

(sugar + yeast + time = ethanol) + (acetic bacteria + oxygen + time) = acid

Part 1: Make Alcohol from Juice

This first vinegar-making method starts with turning fruit juice or some other sweet unfermented juice or liquid into alcohol. If you already have alcohol, you can jump in at Part 2 (page 76).

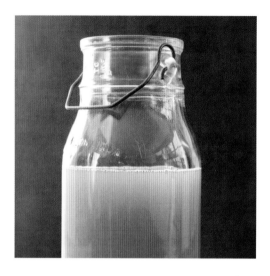

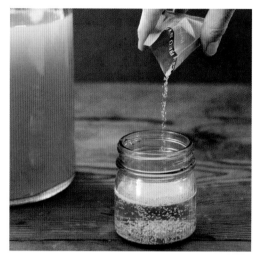

1. If you are measuring, check the sugar content of your juice. Adjust as necessary. Pour room-temperature juice into a clean widemouthed jar. If using spontaneous fermentation, skip to step 7. If using a wild yeast starter, skip to step 5.

2. Add the active dry yeast to unchlorinated water that has been heated to 104°F/40°C.

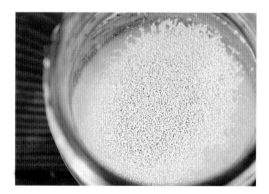

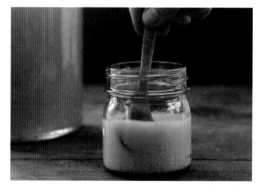

3. Allow the yeast to acclimate on the surface of the water for 20 minutes.

4. Stir the yeasts into the warm water until fully incorporated, then wait for 30 minutes.

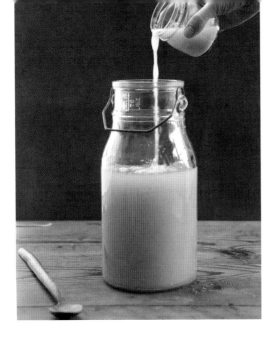

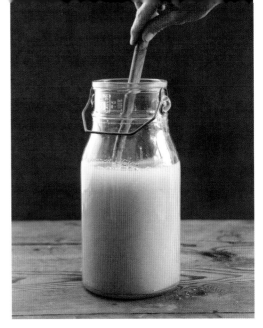

5. Pour the hydrated yeast mixture into the room-temperature juice. Alternatively, pour the wild yeast starter (as made on page 53) into the juice.

6. Stir to incorporate.

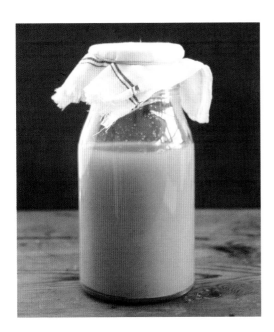

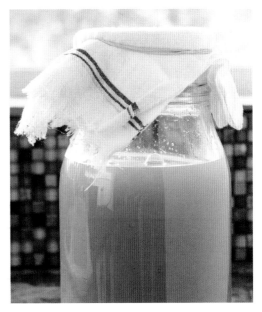

7. Place an air-permeable top, cloth, or coffee filter on the jar and fasten a rubber band or string around it to keep it in place.

8. Ferment for at least 7 to 14 days, to let the alcohol develop.

Part 2: Make Vinegar from Alcohol

Use either your own homemade alcohol or purchased alcohol for this next sequence. The key is to make sure that alcohol levels above 9 percent ABV are diluted with water and that sulfites are removed (see page 43). There is no need to pasteurize to kill any remaining yeasts.

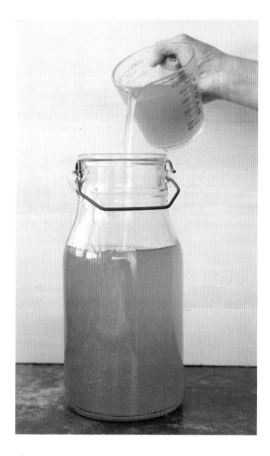

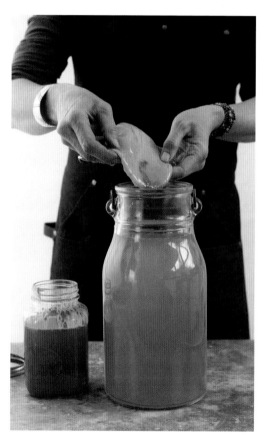

1. Pour the alcohol into your vinegar-making vessel, leaving room for the raw vinegar starter. Add raw (unpasteurized) vinegar for the backslop if no mother is available. Use a ratio of 20 percent of the volume of the cider.

2. If you have a mother that is 4 to 5 ounces (115 to 140 g) per gallon (3785 mL) of cider, or a piece that will cover at least 30 percent of the surface, add the mother with the vinegar that it comes in if purchased or storing. Try to place the mother so that it floats, but don't worry if it doesn't.

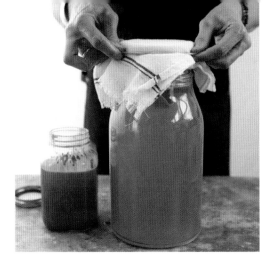
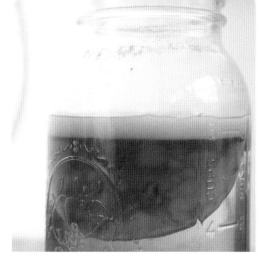

3. Cover the jar with a piece of cloth or a coffee filter to keep out fruit flies. Secure it with a string, rubber band, or the band from the jar over the cloth or filter. Place out of the way in a spot that is 75° to 86°F/25° to 30°C.

4. Check every few weeks. If a mother forms on the surface, it will look very thin, wispy, and translucent at first. Try not to knock the jar, and there is no need to stir—you don't want the new mother to sink.

5. After the mother has formed, the vinegar can continue to age for at least a month or two in a cooler place.

6. After 2 to 4 months, test the pH: It should be 4.0 or lower. You can carefully remove the mother and bottle it. At this point, the vinegar is stable. You can use it immediately or age it. The flavor will mellow with aging.

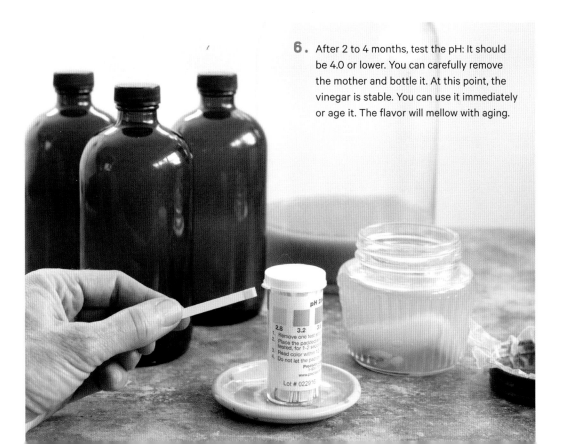

Making Vinegar from Fruit or Vegetable Scraps or Mash

This method uses peels, cores, or other scraps from fruits or vegetables. This can mean taking advantage of what you have at the moment or saving and freezing the scraps (asparagus ends, for example) until you have enough. This is also the method for using the pomace from pressing apples or pears or for making a mash with fresh fruit; it's the classic way many fruit wines are produced. With this method, you can allow wild fermentation, which means utilizing the yeasts that are naturally occurring on the fruit. Alternatively, you can pitch in the yeast of your choice—either a commercial yeast or wild botanical starter.

If your fruit scraps have enough sugar in them, you can simply add raw vinegar when the water in the recipe that follows cools to room temperature. Chances are that your scraps won't quite have enough sugar, though. If you don't want to measure their sugar content, you can add a blanket amount of ⅔ cup (75 g) sugar per quart (946 mL) of water. However, your success rates will increase significantly if you take a sugar measurement and add as much sugar as is needed to achieve at least a 5 percent ABV.

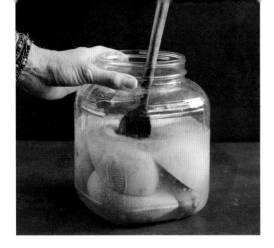

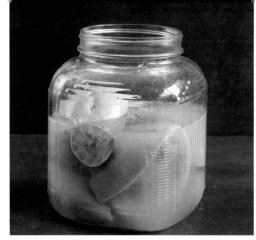

1. Fill a jar with at least a pound of fruit (scraps or mashed fresh). Fill to the neck of the jar with hot, just-boiled, unchlorinated water. Stir well. Allow to sit for 24 hours, then add sugar.

2. Either use the blanket amount above or measure the sugar content of the liquid. To do this, strain some of the liquid and take a specific gravity or Brix reading to determine ABV. See pages 55–59 for detailed instructions. To produce a 5 percent alcohol, the SG should be 1.038. For about a 1 percent increase in ABV, you should add 5 ½ teaspoons (23 g) of sugar to every quart (946 mL) of juice. Add the optional yeast at this point.

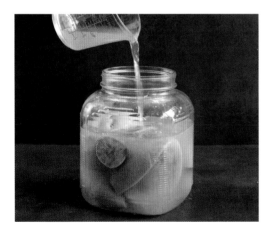

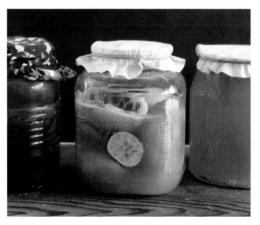

3. In most cases allow to ferment for a week before adding the vinegar. Add raw, unpasteurized vinegar, using 1 cup (237 mL) per quart (946 mL) of water added. Stir well with a wooden spoon. Unlike with most ferments, you want to get some oxygen in the mix. However, make sure the fruit scraps themselves stay submerged, otherwise they can become a host for undesirable opportunistic bacteria.

4. Cover the jar with a piece of unbleached cotton (butter muslin or tightly woven cheesecloth), or a basket-style paper coffee filter. Secure with a string, rubber band, or a metal jar band. Place on your counter or in another spot that is 75° to 86°F/25° to 30°C. Remove the cover and stir with a wooden spoon once a day for the first 5 or 6 days, and occasionally thereafter. You may begin to see bubbles—that's good.

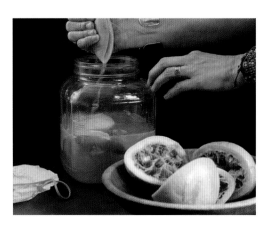

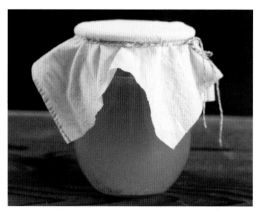

5. In about 2 weeks, the ferment will begin to slow down, and it will be time to take out the scraps. When you remove the cover, you may see a film developing on top of the fruit; this is the beginning of the vinegar mother. Remove and set it aside while you're straining out the fruit solids.

6. Transfer the almost-vinegar (and the MOV, if you have one) to a clean jar and cover again.

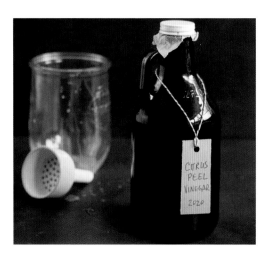

GIVE US THIS DAY OUR DAILY STIR

Fermenting vinegar loves oxygen. Often at the beginning of a batch, especially if there are chunks of fruit, or a slurry of mashed fruits or grains, you'll want to give the mixture a quick stir every day with a wooden spoon. This will get oxygen down deep, feeding the microbes that need it to do their work. I rarely stir batches that are all liquid, unless they are growing surface yeasts; stirring will disrupt the yeast by drowning it. If a mother is forming, I leave it alone so that it can expand across the surface and offer protection from those pesky surface yeasts. If you prefer not to allow the mother to grow, keep stirring. The recipes that follow will indicate when it's necessary to stir. However, any vinegar can be stirred to speed up the process or avoid surface yeast, as needed.

7. Check the vinegar in a month, when you should have nice acidity. However, it may take another month or two to fully develop. The pH should be 4.0 or below. Bottle the finished vinegar, saving the mother for another batch or for sharing with a friend.

Simultaneous Vinegar Fermentation

With this method, you simultaneously create the alcohol and vinegar. In general, it is preferable to give the yeast a week to get started. There are, however, a few cases where I've found it's better to add the yeast (to begin converting the sugars) and the vinegar mother (who will be waiting for the ethanol) at the same time. Don't worry; they'll work it out.

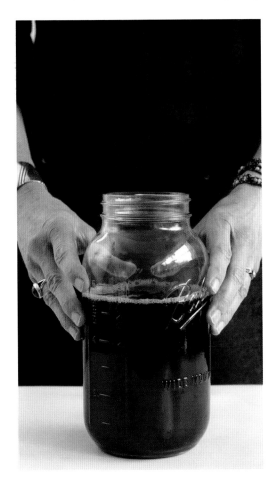

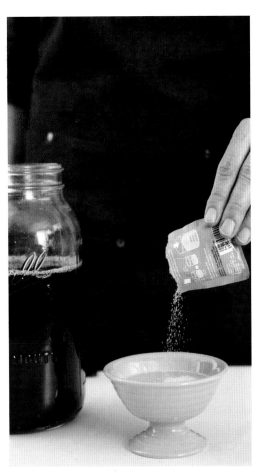

1. Pour room-temperature cider or juice into a widemouthed jar, leaving enough room to add the amount of vinegar, or the mother and the vinegar she comes with, needed for the recipe.

2. Add the active dry yeasts to unchlorinated water that has been heated to 104°F/40°C.

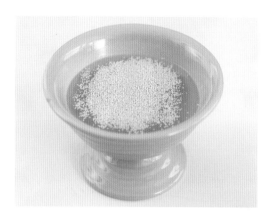

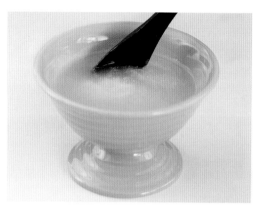

3. Allow the yeast to acclimate on the surface of the water for 15 minutes.

4. Stir the yeasts into the warm water until fully incorporated, then wait for 30 minutes.

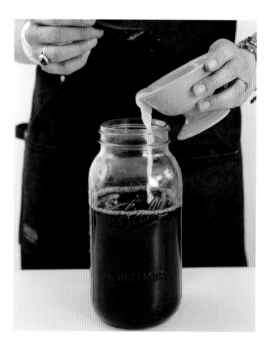

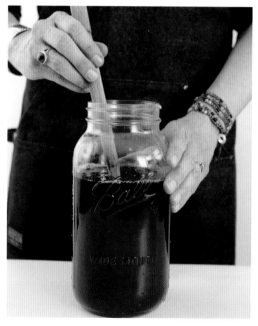

5. Pour the hydrated yeast mixture into the room-temperature juice.

6. Stir to incorporate.

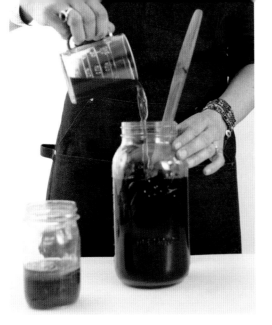

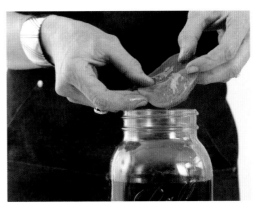

7A. Pour the vinegar starter into the juice. Stir gently; the bacteria are a little sensitive.

7B. Optional step: If you have a mother, place it on top when the juice settles and is still. Sometimes the mother will float, which is ideal, but don't worry if it doesn't.

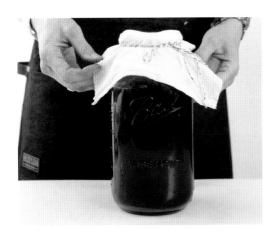

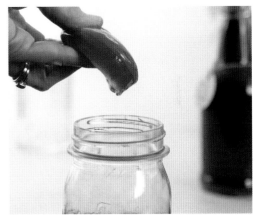

8. Cover the jar with a piece of cloth or a coffee filter. Secure with a string or rubber band, or the band from the jar over the cloth or filter. Place out of the way in a spot that is 75° to 86°F/25° to 30°C. Feel free to check every few weeks. If there is a mother growing on the surface, it will look very thin, wispy, and translucent at first. Try not to knock the jar, and there is no need to stir—you don't want the new mother to sink.

9. After the mother has formed, the vinegar can continue to age for at least 1 or 2 months or longer in a cooler place. After 2 to 4 months, you can carefully remove the mother and bottle it. At this point, the vinegar is stable. You can use it immediately or age it. The flavor will mellow with aging.

FREEING THE SUGAR: STARCH-BASED VINEGARS

The sugars in starchy cereals or tubers—corn, wheat, barley, millet, rice, sweet potatoes, and so on—need to be unlocked. You need an enzyme like alpha-amylase to make the sugar accessible to the yeasts, so that the yeasts can get to work. Think of enzymes as little kids with little scissors cutting a piece of paper into confetti pieces. Enzymes are doing the same, cutting the larger starch molecules into smaller simple sugars.

Historically, depending on when and where you lived, you found a way to get those enzymes working for you. In ancient Egypt and Mesopotamia, early beer brewers figured out germinating grains began this much-needed enzymatic breaking-down process. This technology moved through place and time; in Europe and North America, this is what we now call malting. While I won't be teaching you to malt, in this book you'll learn to make beer vinegar (page 133), which all starts with malting.

In Africa, Asia, and the Americas, people turned to technology as old as, well, saliva, which contains amylases to break down that starch. Chewing and then spitting out the grains inoculated them: voilà, fermentation could begin. Corn chicha, a pre-Columbian corn beer, probably gets the most attention in the US as a beverage made this way.

THE FOUR STEPS OF FERMENTING STARCH-BASED VINEGARS USING KOJI

FIRST FERMENT

Make koji rice. Soak and steam rice, then inoculate it with koji spores and incubate it.

SECOND FERMENT

Free the sugar. Mix koji rice with cooked starch. Enzymes from the koji will release the simple sugars in the cooked starch.

THIRD FERMENT

Ferment the sugar into alcohol. Add yeast to the starch, aerate the mixture, and put it in a fermentation vessel.

FOURTH FERMENT

Acidify the alcohol. Add starter vinegar to the alcoholic mash and allow to acidify. Strain and clarify the cloudy vinegar, then age to smooth the acidity and deepen the flavor.

Koji

Malting has a long history in Asia, but the principal method to release sugar uses mold and yeast. It began in China using *qu* (pronounced *choo*), a starter made of various strains of mold, yeast, and bacteria. Over time, it moved across regions and cultures, and morphed along the way. Some examples are *nuruk* in Korea, *mochi kouji* in Myanmar, and *paeng* in Laos. Methods made their way to Japan in the fourth century CE, and now koji (*Aspergillus oryzae*) is the force behind Japanese vinegar fermentation. Koji mold, a filamentous fungus, secretes enzymes when tasked to grow on starchy mediums, from sweet potatoes to rice. These traditional vinegars are amazing: their history, the processes, and the rich incredible flavors. In this book, you will not be making the traditional distinctive varieties that developed across many regions, but you can learn how to use koji to unlock the flavor treasures bound up in any starch. Instructions for growing koji are on page 277. Going through this process definitely gives one a sense of how much interaction with time, microbes, and ingredients must take place for this final amalgamation of flavor. If you consider the time to grow and harvest the crop, a drop of vinegar is years in the making.

Amazake: Meet the Method

Amazake is a Japanese sweet, aromatically rich rice mash or—more commonly—beverage. Its name translates as "sweet sake." Amazake gains its sweetness from the natural process of the koji breaking down starches into their simple sugars. It is the first step to further fermentation into rice wine, or sake. In this book, think of

WHAT IS BLACK VINEGAR?

The term *black vinegar* refers to long-aged dark vinegars from China and Japan. Although different, balsamic vinegar is the closest comparison, in that these vinegars are deep, rich, mellow, complex, and lightly sweet. The flavors include the umami added by the amino acids that are developed through the fermentation. This long aging also deepens the color, hence the "black" label. This long period of aging develops not only flavor but also many nutritional compounds. As a result, these vinegars are considered extremely healthful.

China and Japan both have myriad regional black vinegar styles. Some are now more widely available, but some are traditional styles that still aren't known outside their region of origin. It is my hope that these ancient practices will continue, but the reality is that many of them are winking out with the older generations.

In Japan, black vinegars are rice based. The most well-known type is called *karosu* and uses brown rice instead of the polished white rice base of regular rice vinegar. In China, most black vinegars are also rice based, but many styles are made with other grains; the many Chinese varieties reflect a wide, nuanced range of ingredients and processes. The type that is known throughout the world as Chinese black vinegar is *zhenjiang*. The common thread among all these styles of black vinegar, besides the long aging, is that the sugar is broken down by mold fermentation—*koji* in Japan and *qu* in China.

amazake making as a technique to access sugars in something and take them on to vinegar. You will combine a cooked starch—grain or starchy veggies like sweet potatoes or winter squash—with koji and provide an environment for the enzymes to do their work, making a mash that you will take on to vinegar.

If you have set up an incubator for other ferments and can reliably set your temperature to that range between 135° and 138°F/57° and 59°C, use that. If you are looking to make amazake but have not yet committed to an incubation setup, here are a few simple alternatives.

OVEN. Some ovens have a setting that allows for a long, slow cook. If your oven does, try it. Just be sure to keep a thermometer in the amazake mixture and check the temperature frequently to ensure it stays in the right range. Once you have dialed in the settings and can trust your setup, you are free to forget about it for a few hours.

CABINET DEHYDRATOR. This appliance works quite well. Remove trays as needed for the size of your jar. Place the jar on the lower rack and set the temperature to 135°F/57°C.

SOUS VIDE METHOD. If you have a sous vide system, place the koji and cooked rice or other starch in a sealed canning jar immersed to just under the lid, or seal the koji and cooked rice in a plastic bag and immerse, with the immersion circulator set to 138°F/59°F.

MULTICOOKER. How you use it depends on what settings your particular model has. Many have a "keep warm" mode that is too warm—145° to 172°F /63° to 78°C—and a yogurt setting that is too low. If your pot has temperature controls, it is a great tool. Set to a range of 135° to 138°F/57° to 59°C. Some cookers have a setting for the Chinese sweet glutinous rice ferment *jiu niang*—95°F/35°C. If you make *jiu niang*, it can be used in place of amazake in recipes. If you have a cooker with a manual temperature setting, then you have the versatility to work with it as you need.

UNDERSTANDING TEMPERATURES

If you grow your own koji as described on page 277, you may notice that amazake is incubated at 138°F/59°C, but koji is incubated between 80° and 95°F/27° and 35°C. This begs the question: How does the koji fungus survive the higher temperature during amazake preparation?

It doesn't. There are two processes at work, with different functions. The first is the growth of the koji mycelium on the cooked rice or other starch; this growth produces the enzymes. After you grow the koji, you are basically harvesting the enzymes to work at breaking down the next substrate, whether it is beans in miso, more grains in amazake or sake, or meats to tenderize. The fungus (spores and mycelium) can't survive above around 113°F/45°C, but the enzymes can persist up to 140°F/60°C.

If amazake is fermented at lower temperatures, say 90° to 100°F/32° to 38°C, the enzymes will work much more slowly. In this situation, lactic acid bacteria will often move in and begin the souring process before the amazake has had a chance to get sweet enough.

Making an Amazake Mash

Amazake is a wonderful tool for making many unique starch-based vinegars. Don't be intimidated by the process; for the sake of simplicity, you'll use premade, purchased koji rice or barley (see Resources, page 285) to add to any starch you choose. It is quick and easy—I promise. And discovering the hidden sugars in these ingredients is magical!

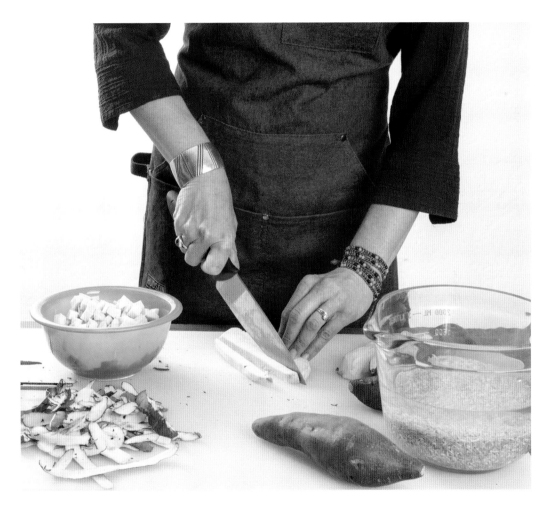

1. If you are making amazake with a whole grain, soak it overnight. If using a starchy tuber or other starch, peel and dice it.

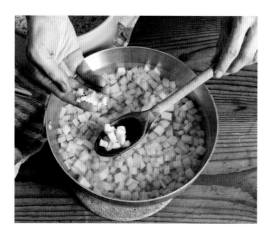

2. Cook your grain or starch until al dente.

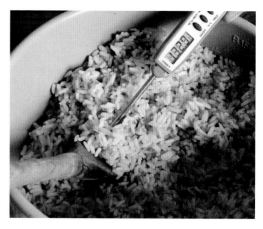

3. Let the starch cool to 135°F/57°C.

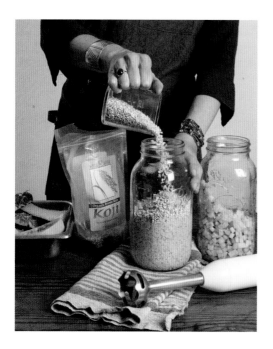

4. Add the koji to the starch, along with any optional fruit scraps.

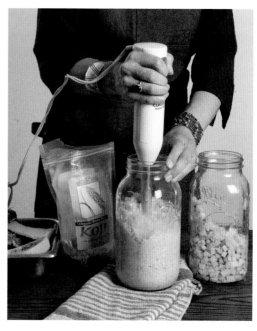

5. Blend to incorporate.

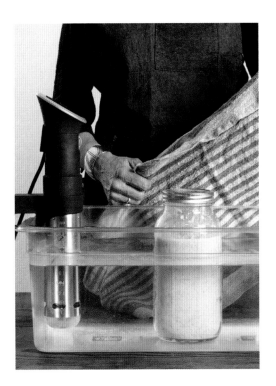
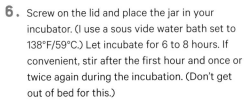

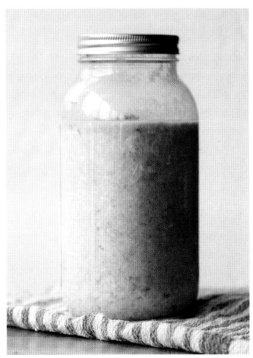

6. Screw on the lid and place the jar in your incubator. (I use a sous vide water bath set to 138°F/59°C.) Let incubate for 6 to 8 hours. If convenient, stir after the first hour and once or twice again during the incubation. (Don't get out of bed for this.)

7. When it cools to 90°F/32°C, add any optional yeast and vinegar starter according to the recipe. Cover with a coffee filter, secured with a rubber band, and place in a spot that is 75° to 86°F/25° to 30°C and convenient for stirring daily for the first 2 to 3 weeks. When finished, the amazake will be liquidy and have a sweet aroma and taste.

Setting Up a Continuous-Brew Vinegar Pot

Setting up a vinegar pot is less about following a particular recipe and more of a lifestyle choice. It can be done in any jar, a ceramic crock, or a wooden open-top pot with a spigot at the bottom. Once you get it going, any remnants of your favorite evening brew or spirit from a can or bottle go into the top of the pot at the end of the evening (or the next morning); out the spigot comes vinegar to be used as needed.

The idea is that the brew in the pot is always fermenting. You can have a white wine and a red wine pot, a beer pot, and a cider pot. Or you can mix and match and prepare your own house vinegar blend. *Note:* I generally like to keep beer with beer, but I often combine cider and wines in one pot.

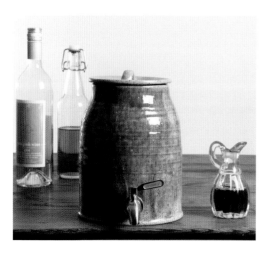
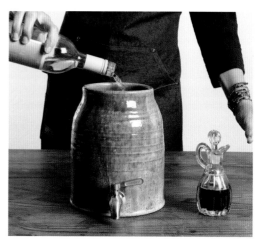

1. Decide what your base alcohol will be and choose a vessel with a spigot on the bottom. Sanitize the vessel by washing in hot, soapy water and air-dry.

2. Pour your starter wine, beer, cider, or other beverage into the vessel. If using wine, check the label for sulfites. If present, treat as described on page 43. Dilute the wine (or any beer or cider that is above 10 percent ABV) with water at a ratio of three parts wine to one part water.

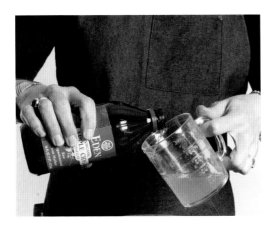

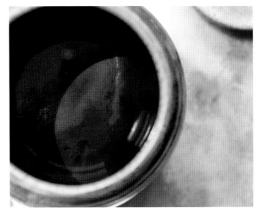

3. Add one part raw vinegar for every four parts alcohol. Cover the pot. Allow a few days for the microbial community to adjust. After about a week, add leftover alcohol as it becomes available.

Note: After this pot is established, you do not need to dilute new additions of alcohol, as it will be automatically diluted by going into the already fermenting pot.

4. After a few weeks, feel free to taste the vinegar, as you desire. After the first 4 to 6 weeks, you can harvest a quantity to bottle, if desired. When the pot is established, you can harvest vinegar followed by adding some new alcohol. Always keep about one-quarter of your container full of the base liquid.

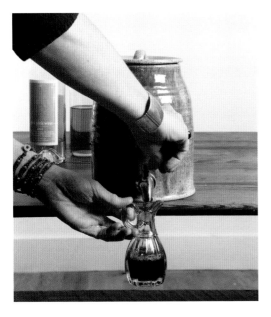

5. If you decide to bottle some of the vinegar, be sure to leave at least one-quarter of the base liquid in the container. For wooden barrels, it's best if you can add some new alcohol at that point, in order to keep the barrel around three-quarters full and keep the staves hydrated. You can do this without disturbing the mother by carefully slipping a tube attached to a funnel alongside the mother. In a ceramic pot, it will be floating. In a wooden barrel, chances are the mother will be stuck to the sides of the vessel and sagging, creating air space over the liquid. If you don't have enough alcohol to fully fill this air space, it's important to loosen the mother at the edges so that it is on top of the liquid. Or remove the mother altogether; otherwise it will dry out and die, and will often mold.

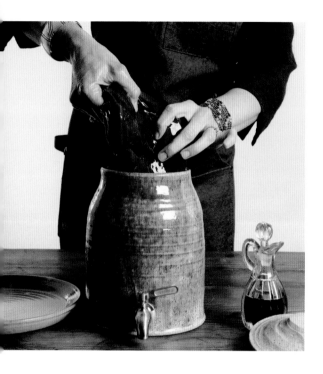

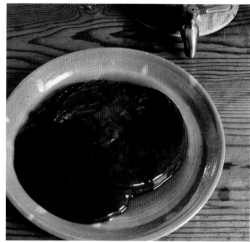

6. Over time—perhaps months or a year or more—the MOV can get very large, or it can fall and clog the spigot. If this happens, just pull out the MOV. As long as there is base liquid, your pot will keep functioning perfectly.

GENERATOR METHODS FOR MAKING VINEGAR

Many people feel that the hardest part about fermentation is the wait. That said, with so much of our food being premade, premixed, and precooked, it is this anticipation that is grounding. Patience is a rare quality these days, though I suspect that humans have always tried to speed things up.

In the seventeenth century, folks were already trying to find new ways to make vinegar faster than it could be created by leaving alcoholic liquid in an open vessel. The Boerhaave process was one of these innovations. It introduced bacteria onto filler materials, such as vines or stalks, which increased the amount of surface area that could come into contact with the bacteria. It also involved moving the liquid frequently to consistently reintroduce oxygen. Similar methods used filler materials (often wood shavings) and some method of movement and introducing air, like rolling the barrel (people power) or rotating barrels (motor powered).

Schuzenbach's quick vinegar process and the Frings generator both rely on dripping the alcohol through the filler materials while blowing in fresh air. The Frings generator keeps the bacteria submerged. It is a stainless steel tank with internal coils, where oxygen is blown directly into the alcohol—so much air, in fact, that it can produce a much higher acid vinegar. Once the alcohol level has dropped to below 0.3 percent, a third of the vinegar is drained off and new alcohol is added. In this way, generators create a continuous brew. Variations of these generators and the Frings Acetator are still in use by some artisans but can require quite a bit of setup and capital.

Modified Generators

In the pages that follow, I will share two simple, small-scale methods for vinegar generators.

KITCHEN-COUNTER BOERHAAVE METHOD. This first method is a nod to old-school production. You and two jars in your kitchen become the generator; this is as off the grid as the seventeenth century. This process can make vinegar in as few as 10 days. As you will read, the more you move the vinegar from jar to jar, the more oxygen gets in, and the faster the fermentation goes. Depending on the materials selected, this technique can be a powerful tool for flavor because you can use any edible plant material as the packing materials. Want oaky barrel-aged flavors? Try oak chips. Want culinary notes? Add rosemary, fennel, or basil stems, or any other herbal stalk. Want woodsy flavors? Use fir sticks, dried turkey tails, and so on. My favorite Fig Leaf Vinegar on page 127 utilizes this method.

AERATION METHOD. The second method is a less hands-on approach to aerating your vinegar (remember, it's all about oxygen) with an aquarium aerator. The aeration method only speeds up the process; it doesn't enhance flavor. In fact, I find that the vinegars made with this method *lose*

flavor. I think that the volatile flavor compounds hitch a ride right out of the liquid and into the air.

For both techniques, the instructions assume that you're starting with already fermented alcohol that is 5 to 9 percent ABV or has been diluted to be in that range. It doesn't need to be an aged alcohol; usually a 10- to 14-day fermentation is enough to convert your fruit juice into enough alcohol to get started. In other words, these instructions start at the second step of the vinegar's two-step process. (See page 74 for starting vinegar with juice.) These techniques can be used for any of the vinegar recipes in the book that are written as the two-step process. They aren't appropriate for the simultaneous fermentations.

Also, both methods will work with smaller and larger vessels. For the aeration method, the same aerating pump will work in a smaller jar or a larger food-grade bucket. The only thing to remember with the kitchen-counter Boerhaave method is the larger the vessel, the heavier that daily pour will be.

Kitchen-Counter Boerhaave Method

In addition to speeding up the process, this is an interesting way to impart a barrel-aged or herbal flavor to your vinegar without the barrel. In fact, I find this is the best part. And honestly, there is a meditative quality about transferring the fermenting vinegar from jar to jar daily. I find that it works best with half-gallon or gallon jars. You will need some filler material for the two jars; experiment with these, or try the Gin Botanical Spirited Vinegar (page 251) or the Bourbon-Style "Drink"-ing Vinegar (page 249) to start.

It's important that you transfer the vinegar daily, to prevent surface yeast from developing. Once surface yeast moves into the filler materials it is nearly impossible to recover.

Once you have this method set up, you can use it for multiple batches of vinegar. When one batch is done, you simply bottle it and start again with the same materials, which are now fully inoculated with acetic bacteria. It's important that you transfer the vinegar daily, to prevent surface yeast from developing. Once surface yeast moves into the filler materials it is nearly impossible to recover.

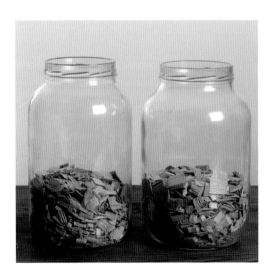

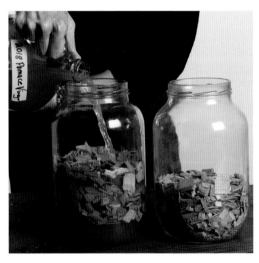

1. Divide the wood chips, herb stalks, or other filler material evenly between two sterilized jars.

2. The filler material should be inoculated and acidified before it can be used in vinegar making. Pour the unpasteurized vinegar over the chips of one jar until they are covered. Let the chips marinate for an hour or two.

NOTE: I find inoculating the material ensures success and speeds up the process. However, the truth is most botanicals, like fennel stalks and fig leaves, will come loaded with wild acetic bacteria, so inoculating is not strictly necessary.

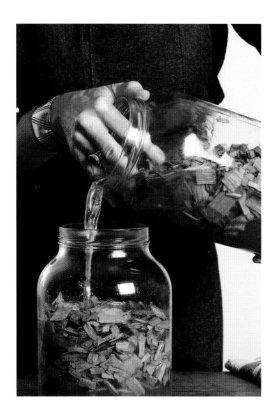

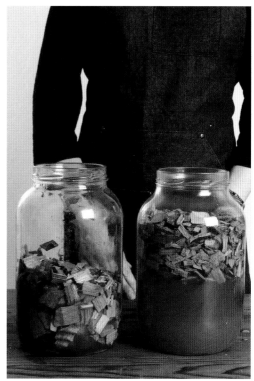

3. Pour off the vinegar into the second jar. Repeat the soaking time. Drain the remaining vinegar (whatever has not been soaked up by the chips) from the second jar, strain it, and bottle it to store or use. Alternatively, you can put the vinegar in one of the jars and it will become part of the new vinegar (though this extra vinegar isn't needed as a starter).

4. At this point, you are ready to add the alcoholic liquid for your future vinegar. Fill one jar to the top with your base alcohol. This will give you the starting amount. Now pour about one-quarter of that into the second jar. This will leave you with one jar that is three-quarters full and another that is one-quarter full.

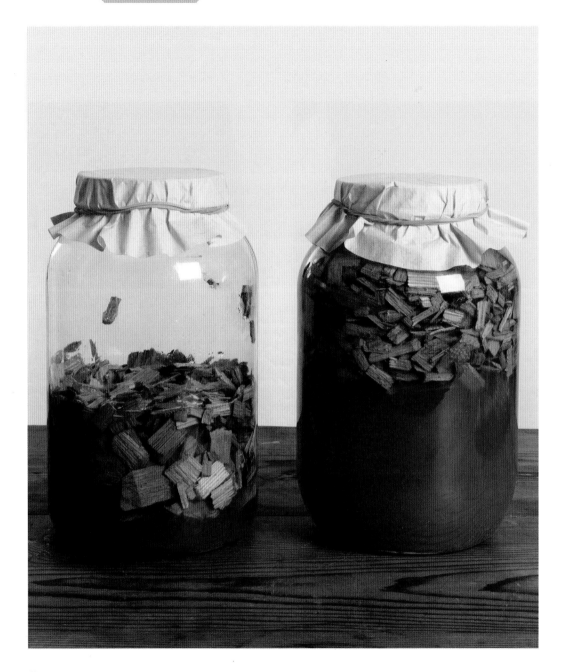

5. Cover both jars with cloth and fasten with a rubber band or string. Place the jars in a spot that is 75° to 86°F/25° to 30°C and convenient to access; you'll be working with it daily. Over the next few days, you'll notice the chips will continue to swell.

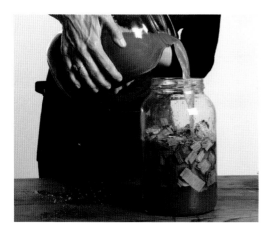 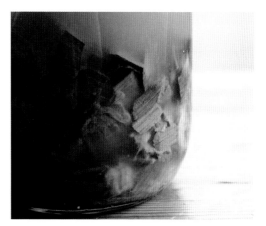

6. The next day, pour the liquid from the nearly full jar into the other jar, leaving about one-quarter in the bottom of the first jar and exposing most of the filler material. This will move oxygen through the liquid and give the bacteria on the filler material time to "breathe." Do this once daily. (You can do it two to three times a day to speed the process.) As the chips swell, add more base alcohol, if needed, to keep one jar full and the other at that quarter mark. In a few days, you will start to smell the distinctive vinegar aroma. Continue to transfer from jar to jar. Assuming you're transferring the liquid daily, in the right temperature range, you will have half-finished vinegar in about 7 days.

7. To finish the vinegar, keep transferring daily. In about 3 weeks, you should have a finished vinegar. After the first round, the process will be faster as the chips are fully inoculated. In fact, at some point you'll see bits of a mother forming on the chips. Traditionally, in larger commercial and artisanal batches, this mother is removed so that it doesn't continue to build up and slow down (or even plug up) systems. If you will be doing many batches, you can either remove the mother or leave it; it won't interfere with the process at this small scale. The bacteria have inoculated your material and will work with or without the mother cellulose.

8. Bottle the finished vinegar. Use immediately or let it age.

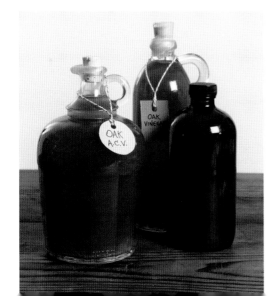

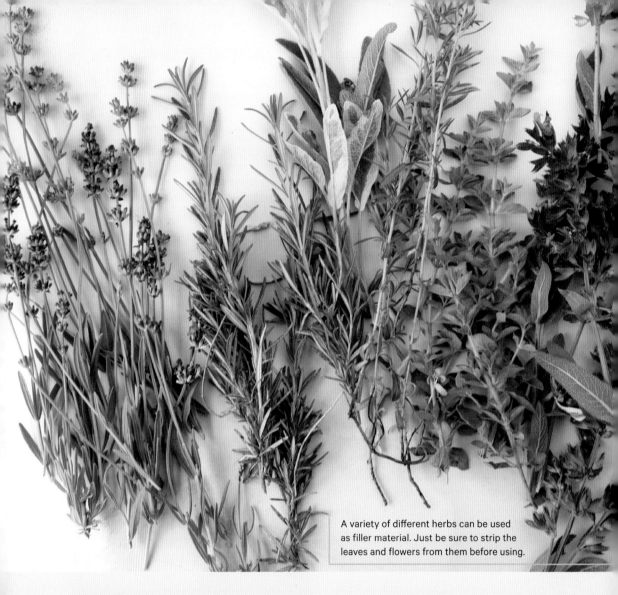

A variety of different herbs can be used as filler material. Just be sure to strip the leaves and flowers from them before using.

TRY THIS:
USE FUN FILLER MATERIALS

Filler materials, also called packing materials, are put in vinegar generators to provide more surface area for the bacteria to live on, as the liquid is drizzled across it. With the simple kitchen-counter Boerhaave method, you will use either organic or inorganic materials to create this surface.

ORGANIC MATERIALS. In the past, grape stalks were often used, since these were easy to procure in wine country. Any type of plant material that is nontoxic is okay to use. In fact, they can add wonderful flavors and compounds to your vinegar as it is brewing. I find that these vinegars have much more depth of flavor than one that has been infused postproduction.

If you have a garden, you can look at what might be available: corn stalks, dried corncobs, fennel stalks, basil stalks, nettle stalks, any herb or spice. In fact, I like to use cut pieces of grapevine, with herbs or spices, not only because we have an abundance but also because the grapevine has a neutral flavor and can tone down herbal flavors that are too strong. Many herbs become slimy and can only be used one time, though I have found that dried herb stalks can be used multiple times. You can use dried fruits, which will render a sweeter, milder vinegar, though they can only be used once. When you're done, these now-acidic fruits can be added to baked goods for a fantastic flavor boost. Dried citrus peels or black lime (known as *loomi*) works well for making delicious drinking vinegars. Wood is easy to source and can add barrel flavors. Cherrywood, applewood, beechwood, medium-char oak chips, and woods or botanicals with resin like fir, cannabis stalks, and so on (as long as they are nontoxic) are also fine but will add very strong flavors.

INORGANIC MATERIALS. These fillers are generally clay or ceramic pieces. They are widely used in small generators because of their long shelf life and neutral flavors and because they produce clear vinegars. I have not used inorganic materials in the simple method outlined in this book, simply because I love the flavors of all the botanicals.

Whether you use organic or inorganic fillers, rinse the chosen material before using it. Most of the fillers I use are aromatic, so this rinse is sufficient for me; boiling them would ruin the delicate flavors. Use your judgment, though. If you're using sticks gathered from the ground, for example, you may want to immerse them in boiling water for 3 to 5 minutes to remove unwanted bacteria.

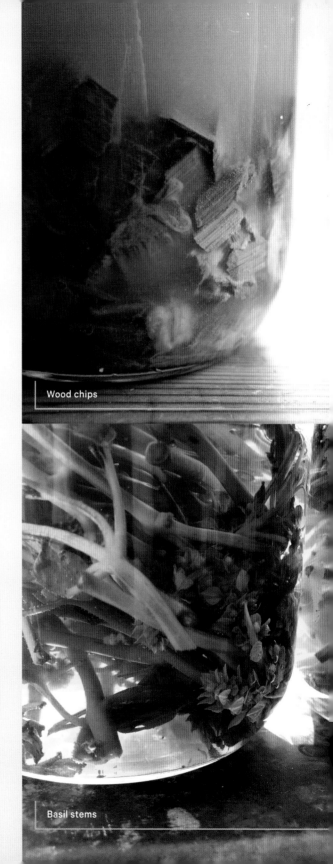

Wood chips

Basil stems

Aeration Method

This method, which starts with alcohol, is the fastest one I present in this book. It simply increases the oxygen available to the bacteria by pumping a little bit in 24/7. It is mechanical; just plug in the aerator and taste the vinegar every few days until it's done. For most vinegar in the right temperature range, this will take 10 to 14 days. As with all newly minted vinegars, it will be ready to use, but aging time will smooth out any harsh flavors. The rub, of course, is that adding the air in this way can compromise flavor.

Here are a few additional tips for making vinegar with this process:

- **TINY BUBBLES ARE BEST.** This is the most important thing to keep in mind. You want very small, gentle bubbles, to avoid losing too much alcohol content to evaporation.

- **LEAVE SOME HEADSPACE.** Use a vessel that gives you a good amount of space at the top, to avoid splattering.

- **USE A FAT MOTHER.** This method doesn't create a mother; there isn't really enough time, and the constant movement makes it difficult for a mother to grow in peace. However, I've found that adding a mother to cap the liquid helps mitigate some of the flavor loss. If you have a thick mother from another batch of vinegar, you can place it on top of the liquid, and it won't be disturbed; the bubbles can keep the MOV buoyant. The air-pump tubing will slip in right alongside the MOV.

- **RIG UP AN AIR DIFFUSER.** You will need a small air pump—the kind used for aquariums—as well as the tubing that comes with it. The air pump may or may not come with a stone aerator, but you will need something to diffuse the air and weigh down the tube. Do your research on materials. I've found that typical aquarium air stones, which are often made of lava, deteriorate in this environment pretty quickly. Others are synthetic resin, and I'm not sure if they are food grade. One option is to crimp the end of the tubing with a small zip tie, then use a needle to prick small holes along the tube for about 2 or 3 inches, starting at the crimped end. You can then place a wooden or glass bead on the tube to keep it from floating.

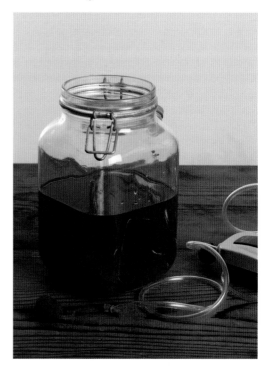

1. Put the base and raw vinegar and/or optional MOV into the jar.

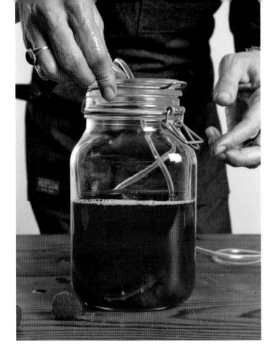

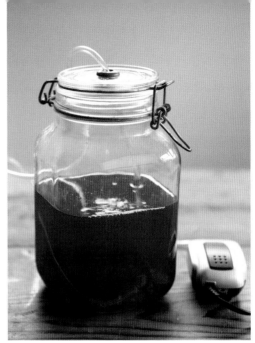

2. Run the tubing with a diffuser on the end (see above) into the liquid.

3. Place the airlock and fasten the lid, or cover with a cloth and fasten with a rubber band or string. Place the jar in a spot in that is 75° to 86°F/25° to 30°C (see page 86 for more specifics on temperature).

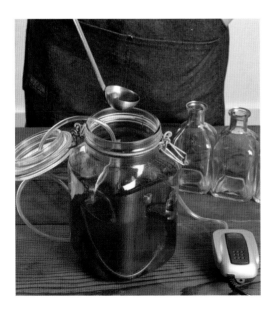

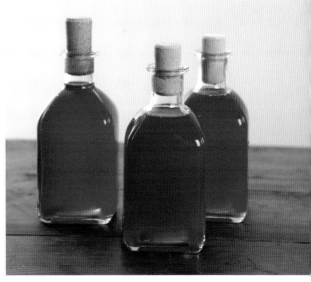

4. Allow to ferment for 10 to 14 days. Check by tasting. If it is ready, you won't taste alcohol; bottle it. If it's not ready, continue to ferment, tasting every few days.

5. Bottle the finished vinegar. Use it immediately or let it age.

FILTERING AND PASTEURIZING

Before you bottle your vinegar, you can consider fine filtering and pasteurizing it. There are many levels of filtering. The first is simply removing large, chunky fruit solids, seeds, or peels. The next level is getting out many of the smaller solids, like hulls from a whole grain vinegar. The final is fine filtering, also called clarifying or fining.

Removing Solids

Why might you want to filter your vinegar? First of all, you might want a clearer vinegar if you'll be giving it as a gift. I have read that clearer vinegars are more stable in storage, but I actually haven't encountered lack of clarity as a storage problem. The solids not only don't bother me, I think they're part of the charm, flavor, and health benefits of homemade vinegar. I do not filter our vinegar. If you'd like to filter yours, here's how to go about it.

RACKING. If your vinegar has been undisturbed, it will be relatively clear, with solids on the bottom. If you have a racking cane (essentially, a type of siphon) for brewing, you can use this to transfer the layer of clear liquid into sanitized bottles. If you don't have a racking cane, any food-grade tubing will also do the trick. If you're careful to keep the cane from touching the bottom, your vinegar will be quite clear. If your vinegar has a mother, you can keep it in a jar with the vinegar that's left with the solids, ready to inoculate your next batch. Be aware that if you're racking directly into bottles, you may see some solids develop, as the last of the bacteria die off and sink to the bottom. It will be minimal, though.

FILTERING. If you don't have a racking cane, or if you want to make sure you capture all the liquid, you can run the vinegar through one or more coffee filters to take out the largest sediment. For finer filtering, use wine filtering papers or kits.

If you want a truly clear vinegar you can investigate the process of fining, which is used in winemaking. It's a process in which a substance (like gelatin) is added to the vinegar and acts like a sponge to bond with the particles in the vinegar. These fining agents can be found at home-brewing suppliers.

STRAINING AND RACKING FOR CLARITY

If my mash (be it fruit based or grain based) is thick, I will hang it in a nut milk straining bag or in a high-quality cheesecloth like butter muslin. The liquid will slowly strain out. Given that vinegar is an oxygen-open fermentation, it can be left many hours without ill effect. Letting gravity and time do this fits my sense of patience. The liquid drips out and the thicker mash turns out of the cloth and is ready for other uses (see page 167). Using a fine-mesh household strainer will remove a lot of the mash. I use a strainer often, especially if the vinegar is fairly thin and I just want to get out the larger particles. Either of these methods will still yield a milky vinegar. This works for me.

Another option is a food strainer—also called a food mill or sauce maker. You can run your thicker vinegar, like a whole-fruit persimmon vinegar or a koji-based vinegar, through it. It will eliminate a lot of the solids but will not fully clarify it.

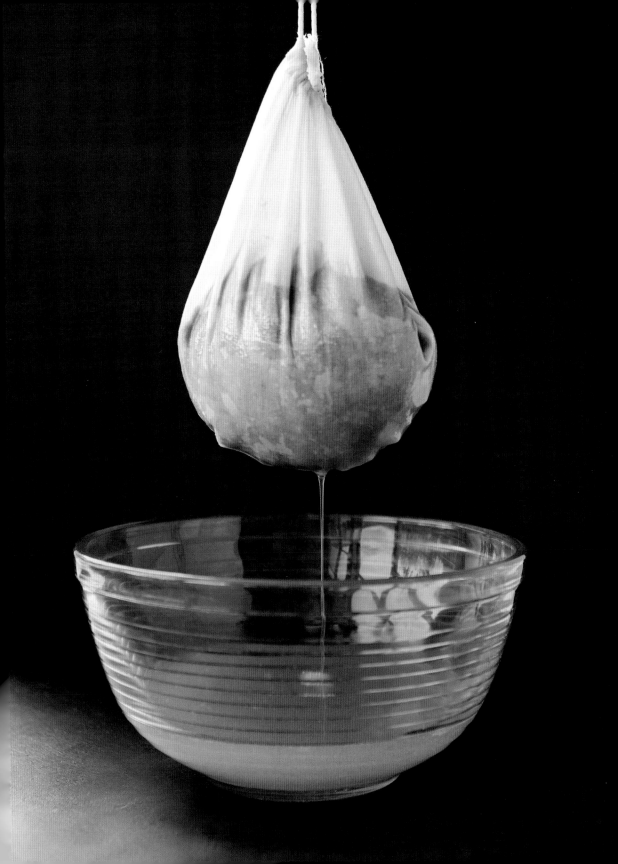

RUSTIC CLOUDY VINEGARS:
CHANGING YOUR PARADIGM

As you will see, koji-based starch vinegars are not a fermenting juice. You are fermenting a thick, acidifying porridge. When the fermentation is complete, the solids are still there. In most cases, they do settle out to the bottom, but this settled mash can still be a significant portion of the contents of your jar. The solution is to rack the clear liquid off the top. You are left with a much smaller amount of vinegar and the lees. In the spirit of whole utilization, there are ideas for using the lees on page 167. That said, I have had a few chats about this very subject with my dear friend, vinegar maker, and koji mentor, Chef Jeremy Umansky, coauthor of *Koji Alchemy*. We invite you to think for a moment about why the vinegar needs to be clear. Sure, commercially available rice vinegars are fined and filtered, giving you clean, clear colors from light yellow to ocher and even deep, dark black. However, if you think about it, clear doesn't make a difference in most vinegar applications. If you are thinking health bennies, then all those little microbes (dead or alive) hanging out in the lees provide nutrition. Jeremy points out that food waste comes from the cultural construct of only one way to use an ingredient (I might add a new one, at that) and what supermarkets have trained us to think food should look like. Once you get past expectations, you will find a thicker, milky vinegar can be sumptuous. It has more body and umami to add to the acidity. When using, just be sure to shake before each pour.

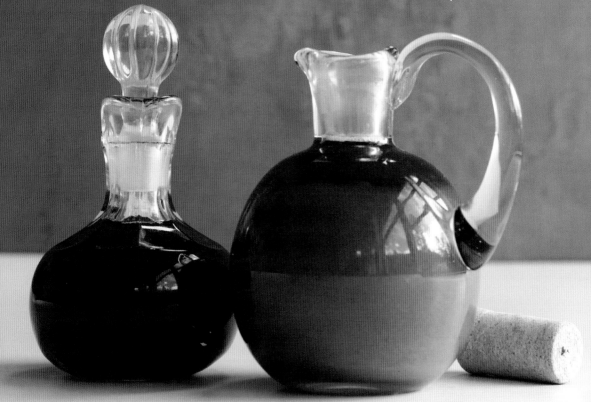

Racking for Clarity

To achieve a clear vinegar, allow the solids to settle out completely. Put your vinegar vessel in the refrigerator (the cold environment will help particles settle), then rack the clear vinegar off the top.

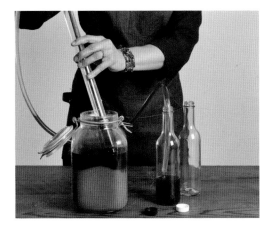

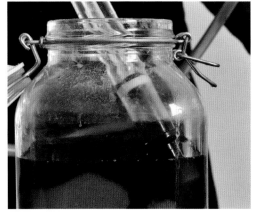

1. Insert a sanitized racking cane into the vinegar, and the end of the tube into an empty bottle. Create suction in the siphon until the tube begins to fill.

2. Monitor the racking cane, being sure to keep it above the lees.

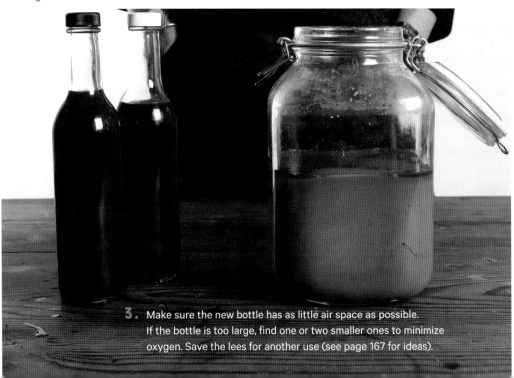

3. Make sure the new bottle has as little air space as possible. If the bottle is too large, find one or two smaller ones to minimize oxygen. Save the lees for another use (see page 167 for ideas).

HOW TO
PASTEURIZE VINEGAR

If you decide to pasteurize your vinegar, you can choose from two methods. The first happens right before bottling. Use a container that is nonreactive, and slowly heat the vinegar over the lowest heat to 140°F/60°C. Hold it at that temperature for around 30 minutes. Since the liquid takes a while to cool, I pull the vinegar off the heat after 20 minutes. I find putting the pot in the oven after I have brought it to temperature on the stovetop helps keep this steady temperature. Avoid heating it above 140°F/60°C, or you will damage the flavors.

An alternative method is to pasteurize the vinegar after it's been bottled. Fill sanitized bottles with vinegar (and any additional ingredients like syrup) to within an inch of the top. Leave the caps off, and set the bottles in a canner or other large pot that has been partially filled with cool water; the water should be at the level of the vinegar. An immersion circulator or sous vide setup works quite well. Heat gently to 140°F/60°C and maintain this temperature for 30 minutes. Carefully remove the bottles from the water, cap, and cool as quickly as possible. To facilitate cooling, you can put the bottles in a cool-water bath and, once they have adjusted to the initial temperature change after a few moments, slowly add ice; you don't want to burst the bottles with a too-rapid temperature change.

Pasteurizing

Pasteurization kills any bacteria and halts further fermentation. Because pasteurization involves heating, and heating compromises flavor and diminishes the health benefits of vinegar, I prefer the raw product. There are only a couple of instances in which I pasteurize our vinegar. One is when I am trying to rid an otherwise-healthy batch of vinegar of a stubborn case of surface yeast. (See Troubleshooting, page 274, for more about that.)

The other time I pasteurize is when I want to back-sweeten a vinegar with honey or a syrup. Unless I pasteurize the vinegar, I'm just feeding the microbes; the yeasts in the "finished" vinegar wake up and begin to ferment anew. That can be fun if you're looking for a lightly alcoholic sparkling vinegar, but not if you're trying to age your vinegar. With pasteurization, you can make sweetened vinegars such as Mead to Honey Vinegar (page 206) or Balsamic-Style Apple Vinegar (page 121).

It's not necessary to pasteurize vinegar to keep it from spoiling; after all, it's so good at inhibiting bacterial growth, it's used to preserve other foods. Commercial vinegars are pasteurized to kill the (friendly) bacteria so they don't make the product cloudy. On a similar note, commercial wine vinegars contain sulfites. These are not left over from the wine itself—they're added to keep the red color in the vinegar. However, we have never experienced our homemade red wine vinegars losing color.

THE HOME STRETCH: BOTTLING AND AGING

How do you know when your vinegar is done fermenting and is ready to be bottled and aged? It's ready when the acidity has developed and the alcohol is mostly gone. I say "mostly" because you certainly won't taste any alcohol, but typically vinegar has a residual 0.3 to 0.5 percent ABV. This is a good thing, as it helps with preservation and is important for developing flavor; the alcohol reacts with the acetic acid to produce aroma compounds (which means it's getting tastier). Home vinegar makers don't really need to worry about testing the alcohol content, but it's important to test the pH; when it's finished, it should be below 4.0 (under 3.7 is even better).

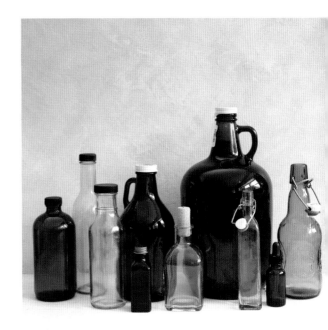

Why Proper Bottling Matters

Once your vinegar is ready, whether you plan to use it immediately or age it, you must remove oxygen from the equation by transferring the vinegar to airtight containers. Otherwise, the acetic bacteria will keep consuming oxygen. When vinegar is exposed to oxygen over a prolonged period, it will eventually become watery. You may see oxidation occur: The vinegar becomes discolored, starting at the top and moving downward over time. (See page 276 for more.) I cannot stress enough how important it is to transfer your vinegar to an airtight container before you begin aging it.

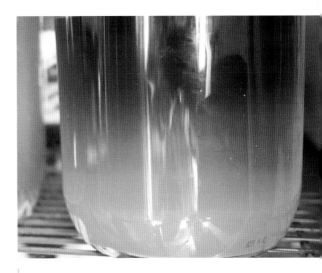

Oxidation can cause vinegar to darken.

WORTHY BOTTLES

Warning: Becoming a vinegar maker will turn you into a bottle saver. The other way to look at it is if you hate to get rid of interesting bottles, you now have a reason to save them. Once you start aging your homemade vinegar, you will never look at bottles the same way.

BOOZE BOTTLES. These can be both unique and beautiful, which is especially nice if you want to give away vinegar. Condiment and sauce bottles with plastic lids are handy, because you don't have to worry about acid corrosion over time. (If you do have a metal lid, simply slip a piece of parchment paper, waxed paper, or waxed cloth in over the top of the bottle before screwing down the lid.)

CORKED BOTTLES. These work well, since they don't corrode. If, as with a bottle of wine, you've bottled in it with a cork that is fully inserted, it will be airtight. This holds true for cork tops with a plastic cap, like you might find on an olive oil bottle. However, I have found that a cork stopper can let in enough oxygen to grow a mother on top of the vinegar in the neck of the bottle. This can be remedied by dipping the top of the stoppered bottle in warm wax to seal it.

AMBER GROWLERS. Kombucha or beer growlers are my favorite bottles for aging. They hold a lot, so when I empty a batch, I can just move it on to aging without thinking about how I will want to bottle the vinegar in a year or more. The vinegars that get used regularly also are convenient to pour from these handled bottles.

BEER AND SODA BOTTLES. I use a lot of bail-top beer and cider bottles, simply because I have a lot of them and they have no drawbacks. I've also used recycled beer bottles that I have capped with a bottle capper for storage or transport. The downside is that you'll need to find another lid or cork once you open a bottle since, unlike beer, vinegar won't be consumed all at once.

CRUETS. These antique table vinegar cruets with glass tops were made to sit on the table alongside salt, pepper, and oil. They're not airtight, so they're best for active use, not storage. I keep a few different vinegar varieties on the table, so that we can add a sprinkle of finishing acid to a dish or splash a bit in our drinking water. I've also found that putting a selection of a half dozen or more vinegars in tincture bottles with droppers is quite enjoyable. Your dinner guests will have fun squirting little drops of scrumptious acid on everything.

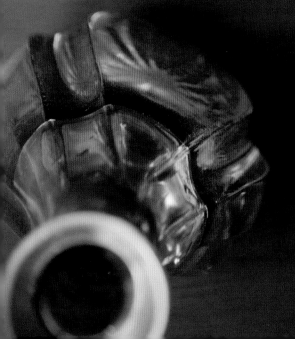
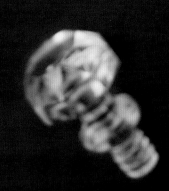

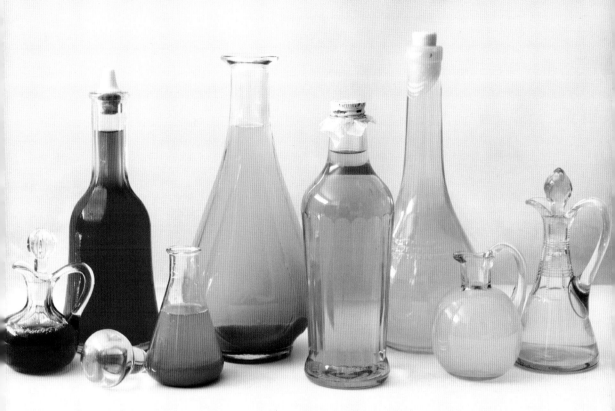

SOUR POWER:
WATCH THOSE LIDS

Here's an extreme example of how corrosive vinegar is. I had some vinegar stored in a mason jar that was deep in the recesses of our fermentation cave, along with all the shelved bottles and jars. When I found it a few years later, the entire middle of the lid was gone, like it had vanished into thin air. Most of the vinegar had evaporated as well.

To avoid this kind of corrosion, I place a sheet of parchment paper between the lid and the vinegar. Unfortunately, most plastic mason jar storage lids are not airtight when used by themselves, so they're not a good option. The only way to make them airtight is to use a silicone sealing ring or food-grade plastic in between the lid and the top of the jar.

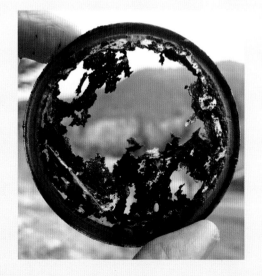

If you have a small quantity of vinegar and can't wait to use some, you may want to use a number of bottles, so that you can use some vinegar soon or after a few months, then age the rest for varying periods of time. Or you can age the entire batch in larger bottles or glass jugs, then transfer it to smaller bottles later. It's best to use narrow-necked bottles and jugs (recycled amber glass kombucha growlers are great) that can be filled to the top; these leave little surface area and minimal air space. I like using pretty, narrow-necked bottles with a plastic cap or a cork for long aging, as these materials won't corrode with the acidity.

I remove the mother when I bottle, but if you want to share part of the mother in the bottle, as a gift for someone to start his or her own batch of vinegar, that's fine. The mother's bacteria won't continue to work without oxygen.

Why Aging Matters

When vinegar is young, it's safe to use but can be strong and harsh. Aging it for at least four to six months will soften the harshness. The amount of time depends on the type of vinegar; corncob vinegar, for example, takes much longer than a fruit-based vinegar. As it sits quietly and ages—find a cool, dark place to store it or use dark-colored bottles, as UV light can be damaging—a lot of things happen with the chemistry. This is when the acids slowly make esters, those delicious flavors you read about on page 28. As the vinegar smooths out, subtle flavors will emerge—maybe ones that were in the fruit, or in the alcohol, and were hiding beneath the blatant acidity. After a few months, alcohol that was left in the liquid will also develop esters that contribute to the flavor. In short, it will get better and better. I have some bottled vinegars that are approaching 10 years old—they are akin to a smooth, aged whiskey.

Barrel Aging

If you're in this for the long haul and have produced a significant quantity of vinegar, you can barrel-age it. It's important for your barrel to be filled to capacity, with no exposed surface area for a new mother to form. Not only will the wood add flavor, but the porousness of the wood will cause the vinegar to evaporate slowly over time. This is how true balsamic is made (see page 112).

One thing to keep in mind is that you need to start with a fairly large quantity of vinegar and plan on moving it to smaller barrels as it ages, because it evaporates. This is what Christopher and I didn't do properly a number of years ago, when we tried this for the first time. We thought we would barrel-age some vinegar for a year or so. We bought a super cute little barrel. It was watertight with no leakage, but there just wasn't enough mass inside—within the year the entire batch had evaporated.

One last small barrel note: Because the ratio of vinegar to surface area of wood is so low, a small, oaky barrel could make the flavor too strong fairly quickly. Taste the vinegar after a few weeks to make sure that it isn't too strong already. If so, you may want to move it to a glass container to continue aging. If it seems fine, taste it again in four or five months.

Small, used barrels can sometimes be procured from distillers. These impart another layer of flavors.

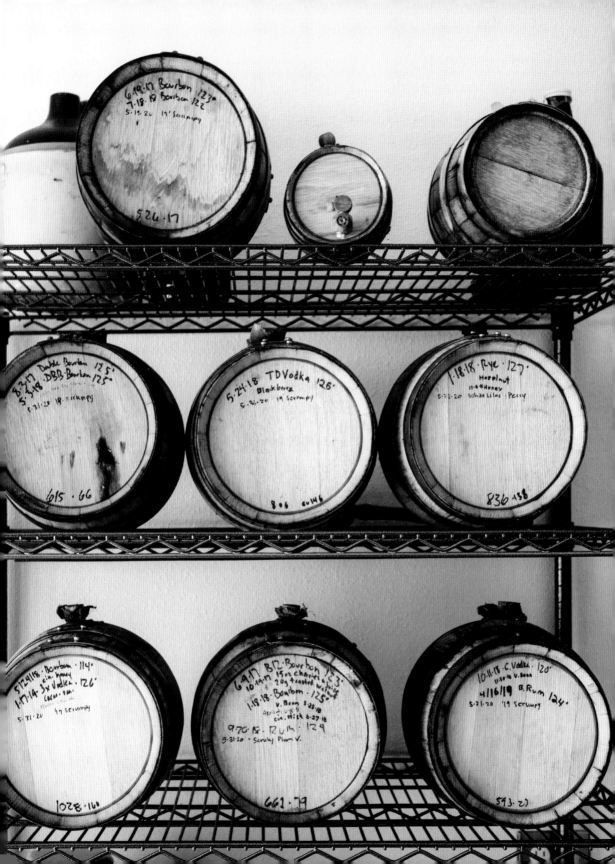

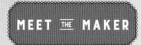

STEVE AND JANE DARLAND,
TRADITIONAL ACETO BALSAMICO OF MONTICELLO

It was only after speaking with Steve and Jane Darland of Traditional Aceto Balsamico of Monticello, in Monticello, New Mexico, that I finally began to understand how true balsamic vinegar is made.

Steve and Jane entered into vinegar making after leaving careers "in tall buildings in San Francisco" to pursue, as they say, something "complicated, hard, delicious, and unique." They refurbished a tumbledown adobe in Monticello, New Mexico, and planted sweet, white Trebbiano and Occhio di Gatto grapes. They ordered casks from Francesco Renzi, whose family has been making top-quality barrels in Modena, Italy, for over five hundred years. Because of the long line of people waiting for barrels, it took nearly three years for the Darlands to get theirs. They have 56 casks, sized from 75 liters down to 10 liters, arranged in sets of seven-cask

batteries with each cask made of a different wood. However, each wood is in a different-sized cask in the different groupings—giving each battery a unique flavor.

JUICING AND FERMENTING

First, though, the grapes must be pressed and the juice fermented. The grapes are picked, run through a crusher/destemmer, and pressed. The juice is set in a cold room, where the pulp settles to the bottom. At this point, the juice is around 23 to 25 degrees Brix. It's racked into 55-gallon stainless steel cookers, where it stays below a simmer for over 70 hours straight, until it reaches the target Brix in the 40s. The temperature is never allowed to exceed 140°F/60°C—too high, and it will begin to candy, and it can't come back from there. The resulting condensed juice goes back into the cold room to sit for a few days. During this time, the juice sets up an undesirable sugar that crystalizes and tastes like sweet alum, which is removed.

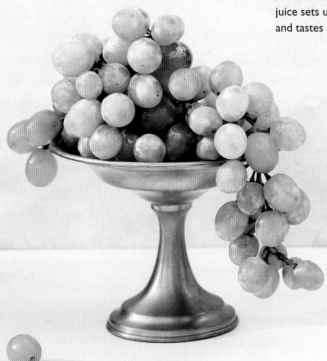

Then it's time to ferment. The *mosto cotto* (cooked must) goes into the fermenters with the yeast *Zygosaccharomyces bailii*, which they get from an Italian-owned lab in Sonoma.

Steve calls it a food-safe bacteria. When I looked it up, I found it's not a bacterium exactly but not a normal brewing yeast either, it is a non-*Saccharomyces* budding yeast. Interestingly, this microbe that is the magic of balsamic is a bugaboo in wine fermentation, where it can be a spoiler. The yeast has a unique ability to tolerate acids and sugars, which are what most foods rely on for preservation, and are exactly what is required for the *mosto cotto* as high sugars and low pH make it a stressful medium for common yeast to grow in. It is also capable of producing more ethyl esters and is a part of other delicious ferments. It is a member of the community in a kombucha SCOBY and is part of the Chinese liquor Maotai, known for containing over three hundred instrumental flavor compounds.[8]

The fermentation starts slowly—sometimes it takes weeks. Steve says that this part makes him anxious; every year, just about the time they feel like it isn't going to start, it does.

After the fermentation period, the hundreds of gallons of resulting wine are inoculated with a mother starter that comes from a mix of vinegar from highly seasoned barrels. At this point, the fermentation comes to a dead stop. It's critical here that the sugar, alcohol, and acidity balance are monitored carefully so after fermentation has reached the low teens of ABV, the sugar is balanced. These food-grade plastic barrels are held cold so that nothing ferments too quickly and so that the particulates can fall out of the liquid and settle on the bottom, in a process called cold fining.

CASK AGING

After this, the *mosto cotto* heads to the first aging barrel and the dense vinegar is hand-pumped into the first cask in a battery. The aging vinegar moves through progressively smaller casks of ash, acacia, chestnut, oak, mulberry, juniper, and cherry, staying in each cask for 1 year. When it is through the first seven, the process starts over, repeating three times for a total of 21 years. When the vinegar makes it through all seven casks in a battery, it goes into the next battery. The Darlands choose the next one based on the taste and where they think it needs to go. Steve describes it as a 21-year process of capturing the flavors of the grapes, the time and place, and the barrels themselves, all in one condensed drop.

Each barrel has an opening that is covered with a cloth, through which everything volatile leaves— water, acetic acid, and alcohol. What is left is the sugar and acid in the main body of the vinegar. The levels of each rise and come into balance with each other.

This process of moving the vinegar is physically demanding, especially as the barrels get smaller and the liquid gets denser—it is slower to pour, and the barrels are heavy. In the Darlands' arid climate, their 21-year balsamic is the equivalent of a 35-year Italian balsamic, according to the established measures defined in Modena by the balsamic consortium. The vinegar to use and sell is only drawn from the smallest barrel, and there is always some vinegar left at the bottom of the barrel to keep the family of vinegar going (think a starter), aptly named patrimony.

Steve and Jane put their first harvest into barrels in 1997. They've carefully managed and mastered the process so well, they were the first non-Italian vinegar makers allowed to enter their traditional balsamic vinegar in Italian competitions.

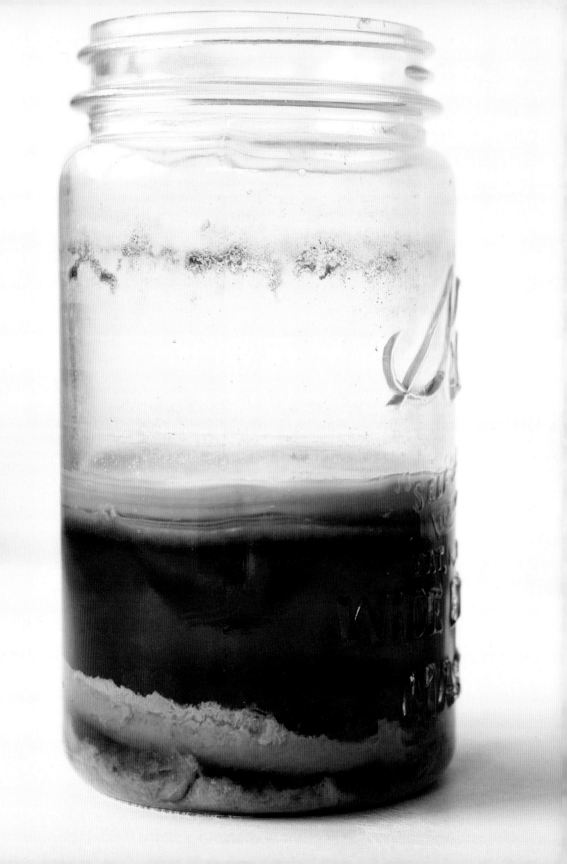

CHAPTER 5

BASIC VINEGARS
FROM CIDER, WINE, AND BEER

As **YOU WELL KNOW** by reading up to this point, to make vinegar you can go completely hands-off and just put the fresh juice in a widemouthed vessel, top it with a cloth, and let time and microbes happen. In my experience, this works perfectly about as often as it does not work at all due to any number of factors—most often harmless but undesirable surface yeasts called kahm yeast, or other unwelcome microbes. These microbes compete for the sugar and nutrients and will cause the process to stall or not happen at all.

In this chapter, the recipes will lead you through making apple, wine, country wine, and beer vinegars that work. Because we all have different preferences, the recipes give options for wild vinegars and yeasted vinegars. I do add a vinegar starter to all of them. While it is not necessary, it helps give the vinegar a good send-off—first by acidifying the liquid, which helps control surface yeasts, and then by seeding it with a good population that goes to work quickly. Of course, if you do not have any way of procuring some unpasteurized vinegar or just want to start with your own populations of acetic bacteria, don't worry: They will move in, and you can then use successful batches for subsequent projects.

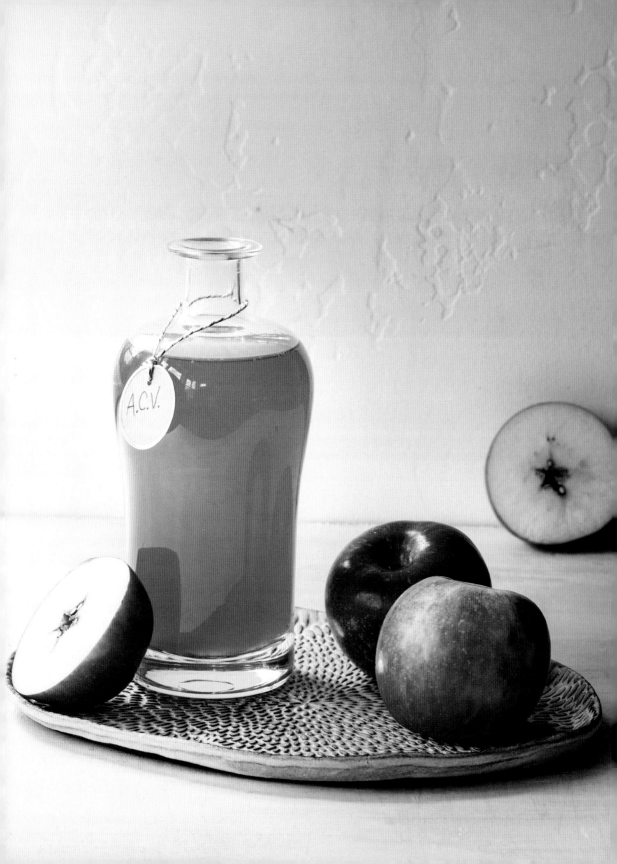

Apple Cider Vinegar

WHY NOT START WITH A CLASSIC? You can make your own delicious ACV, whether you start from your own pressed apple juice, store-bought apple juice, or already fermented hard cider. If you're starting with hard cider, skip to step 5. If you're making it with fresh-pressed juice, you can skip the yeast altogether and do a wild ferment (with flowers, even; see Lilac Vinegar, page 122). If you're starting out with pasteurized juice, you will need yeast. This recipe uses commercial yeast, but you can choose to use a wild yeast starter (see page 53).

Apple juice falls beautifully in the specific gravity range for the perfect alcohol to create a good acidic vinegar. I have never had to adjust with any extra sugar so there isn't a need to measure specific gravity or Brix for successful vinegar, but if you keep a vinegar log and have the tools, you may want to keep track of this. Apples are also naturally acidic fruit. This lower pH means that you won't have to bring the pH down with lemon juice to help get a strong fermentation without surface yeast. This, and most of the recipes in this book don't strictly need a vinegar starter; vinegar will happen on its own. In my years of making vinegar, though, I've found that the success rate is so much higher with the inoculation, there's no reason not to use a starter unless you simply don't have access to raw vinegar.

YIELD
1 gallon

1 gallon (3.8 L) apple juice, freshly pressed or pasteurized (see Note on page 118)

½ teaspoon (1 g) wine yeast (optional for freshly pressed juice, needed for pasteurized juice), hydrated in ¼ cup (59 mL) unchlorinated water, warmed to 104°F/40°C; or ½ cup (118 mL) room-temperature wild yeast starter (page 53)

1 cup (237 mL) raw, unpasteurized, unfiltered vinegar, or a vinegar mother

1. Fill a sanitized 1-gallon jar with juice, leaving about 2 inches of headspace.

2. Add the hydrated yeast or the wild yeast starter to the jar. Alternatively, if wild fermenting, skip to step 4.

3. Cover the jar with a piece of unbleached cotton (butter muslin or tightly woven cheesecloth), or a basket-style coffee filter. Secure with a string, a rubber band, or a threaded metal canning band. This is to keep out fruit flies.

4. Place in an environment where the temperature is between 55° and 65°F/ 13° and 18°C. Wild yeasts seem to do better at this temperature range.

recipe continues on next page

Unlike some active commercial yeasts, wild yeasts are typically slow to start, so don't expect to see bubbles for a couple of days or more. Stop here if you decide you want some hard cider (see the sidebar below).

5. At 7 to 10 days, add the raw vinegar. Replace the cover on the jar. Store on your counter or in another spot that is 75° to 86°F/25° to 30°C.

6. Check the vinegar in a month, when you should have nice acidity. However, it may take an additional month or two to fully develop, especially if your environment is cooler.

7. Bottle the finished vinegar, saving the mother for another batch or sharing with a friend. Use immediately, or age to allow it to mellow and develop flavors.

NOTE: Because this cider is destined to become vinegar, this recipe uses an open container that gives the cider lots of air contact. If you decide you want to drink a bit of the cider and make vinegar with the rest, it's important to use a narrow-mouthed bottle fitted with an airlock during the first fermentation. This recipe is for a gallon, simply because gallon containers are easy to procure. You should feel free to increase or decrease it, as needed. Many ACV recipes online call for cutting apples into chunks and adding sugar and water. While you will get a similar flavor, you will not get the same product. If you want true apple cider vinegar with all its nutrients, you need to start with real apple juice. See page 172 for using leftover pomace after pressing.

WAIT! I WANT SOME HARD CIDER

If you want to have a little hard cider, not just vinegar, you will ferment the apple juice (without adding a vinegar starter) until you no longer see bubbles. At this point, the primary fermentation cycle is likely done. To be sure it's really finished, use a wine thief to draw out a sample and measure the specific gravity. If it's at 1.000 or below, the sugar is gone, and fermentation is complete. If it's

CHASING A
HOMEMADE BALSAMIC

I've been trying to make a balsamic-style apple cider vinegar for a number of years, and some efforts have been better than others. Luckily, after speaking with Steve and Jane Darland (see page 112), I finally got a sense of the actual process. It became obvious why one of my first attempts at making my own ACV balsamic, which consisted of dropping a MOV in a jar of boiled cider without fermenting first, did not work.

Next, I tried dropping a high-sugar-tolerant yeast into a thick, syrupy boiled cider to get the ethanol started. I believe I just sent the yeast to their death. Nothing happened. It was a clear example of why ciders need to be chaptalized (sugar added to raise the resulting ABV; see page 59) when you want to make them with high sugar.

The following year, I used a thinner syrup and fermented it for about three weeks until some of the sugar had turned to ethanol. I then put it in an open jar with a MOV. Meh. It turned into a strong, sparkling ACV, which is not a thing.

Of course, most of the magic is in the aging. Traditional balsamic is aged in a series of progressively smaller barrels made of different woods—chestnut, cherry, mulberry, even juniper—which adds to the complexity of flavor. Before talking to Steve and Jane Darland, I set a mixture of ACV and boiled cider aging in an oak barrel that, as of this writing, has been aging for eight months. It still will never be the real deal, but it might be a tasty and fun slow project.

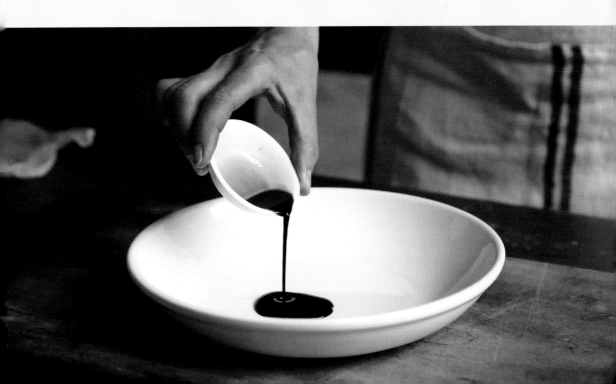

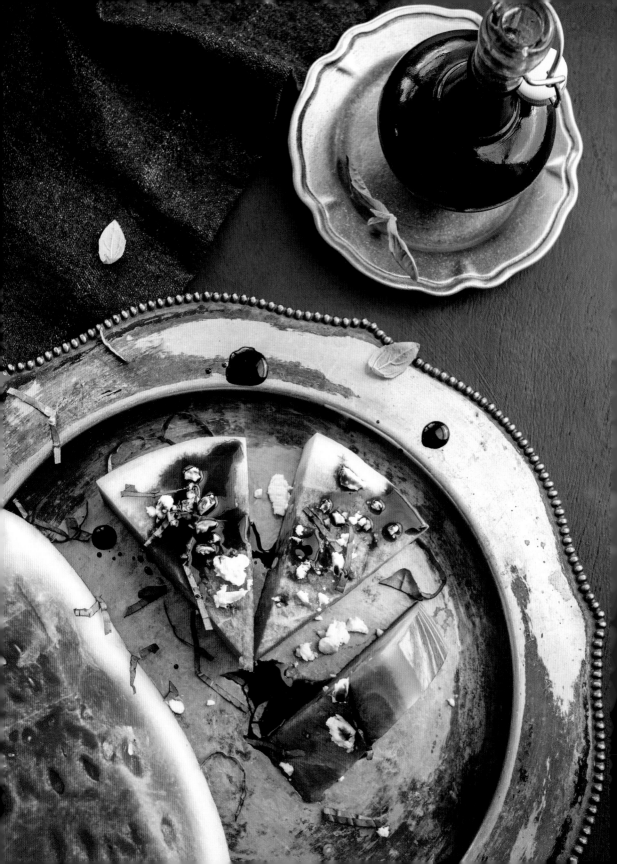

Balsamic-Style Apple Cider Vinegar

I KNOW VERY WELL that I will never make a true balsamic vinegar (and after reading the profile on page 112, you'll understand why). But I also know that its sweet thickness on, say, a wilted bitter greens salad or grilled radicchio makes me crave a homemade substitute. After some experimenting (see Chasing a Homemade Balsamic, page 119), I landed on this recipe, which I'm pleased with. I love that I'm using something we have an abundance of on our homestead—apples—to create something useful and tasty. This version is full-on cheating but has some elements of aged flavor; rich, syrupy texture; and that marriage of sweet and sour—just what we like on our grilled radicchio salads with a little salt and olive oil. Instead of using a barrel to add wood flavors, this recipe uses wood chips or an aging stick. Found at brewing supply stores, aging sticks are often spirals that you can hang in your jar or bottle. Their advantage is that they're easier to remove than chips are. Both options provide as much surface area of wood as possible to the brew. Toasted wood will add more bitter or charred flavors to the wood; untoasted will give more subtle wood flavors.

**YIELD
2–3 cups**

3 cups (710 mL) apple cider vinegar (see Note)

½ cup (28 g) cherry (*Prunus avium*) wood chips, or an aging stick, toasted or untoasted

2½ cups (592 mL) boiled cider (page 238)

1. Combine the vinegar and wood chips in a sanitized half-gallon jar and cover with a lid (you can tighten the lid; there is no fermentation at this stage). Let sit for a day, then taste. The oils and flavors can infuse the vinegar quickly. Let sit until the flavor is pleasing to you; I usually give it 7 to 10 days, then strain out the wood chips. (Save them in a jar for another project or for use with the kitchen-counter Boerhaave method on page 94. If you are not using within a week, freeze until ready to use.)

2. In a stainless steel or other nonreactive saucepan, mix the vinegar and boiled cider.

3. Gently heat to 140°F/60°C to reduce the liquid again. Stir occasionally. When it has reduced to a little less than half of its original amount, or you like it, it is finished.

4. Bottle the finished vinegar. Use immediately or let it age.

NOTE: Alternatively, you can use an apple cider vinegar you have previously made with wood filler material—cherry, oak, chestnut, etc.—by the kitchen-counter Boerhaave method (page 94), in which case start the recipe at step 2.

Lilac Vinegar

BECAUSE OF THEIR EVOCATIVE SCENT in May, lilacs might be the first flower I fell in love with as a wee girl. As an adult, I planted one near a window in each of our yards, wherever we lived. At our home now, a previously planted hedge of them fills the yard. This flower and its scent bring me comfort, and so does the lemony floral vinegar it makes.

This is an apple cider vinegar that has been fermented with the wild yeasts on lilacs. The lilac essence comes through with a sweet floral scent that lingers just above the acidity. The resultant vinegar has a delicate floral quality again within the acidity.

Consider this recipe the base recipe and technique, and see Flower Power: Wild-Fermented Floral Vinegars on page 124 for more ideas.

YIELD
about 1 gallon

1 gallon (3.8 L) pasteurized apple juice

1–2 cups (237–473 mL) lightly packed lilac blossom florets picked from stem clusters

1 cup (237 mL) raw, unpasteurized, unfiltered vinegar, or a vinegar mother

1. Pour most of the juice into a sanitized widemouthed gallon jar, add the blossoms, and pour in as much of the remaining juice as will fit. Stir well with a wooden spoon.

2. Cover the jar with a basket-style coffee filter or a piece of unbleached cotton (butter muslin or tightly woven cheesecloth). Secure with a string, a rubber band, or a threaded metal canning band. This is to keep out fruit flies.

3. If possible, place in an environment where the temperature is between 50° and 65°F/13° and 18°C. Wild yeasts like a cool temperature, so the closer you stay in this range, the better. Wild yeasts typically are slow to start, so don't expect to see bubbles in your jar for a couple of days or more.

4. Stir once a day for the first 5 or 6 days. Unlike with most ferments, you want to get some oxygen in the mix. However, make sure the flower petals themselves stay submerged, otherwise they can become a host for undesirable opportunistic bacteria.

5. Add the raw vinegar. Stir well and replace the covering.

6. Place on your counter or in another spot that is 75° to 86°F/25° to 30°C.

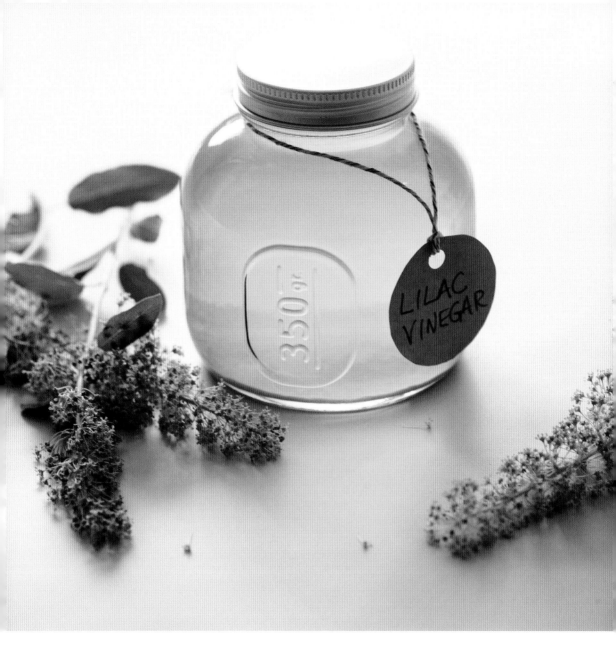

7. Check the vinegar in a month, when you should have nice acidity. However, it may take another month or two to fully develop, especially if your environment is cooler.

8. Bottle the finished vinegar, saving the mother for another batch or sharing with a friend. Use immediately, or age to allow it to mellow and flavors to develop.

FLOWER POWER:
WILD-FERMENTED FLORAL VINEGARS

You can harness wild blossom and botanical yeasts from domesticated plants in your garden or from foraged blossoms. Each blossom vinegar has its own spirit and quality. Because I make a lot of these, I have the luxury of comparing them side by side and have found that they are truly individuals. Dandelion blossoms yield a delicious, mellow, and refreshing vinegar. Sage blossoms produce a savory herbal vinegar that has a floral hint of sage yet doesn't remind you of roasted poultry with stuffing. And manzanita blossoms give the brew rich cinnamon and honey notes: I would have never guessed. Wherever you procure your blossoms, be sure that they are edible and unsprayed; you want those yeasts alive and well, and you don't want to add unknown chemical pollutants to the mix.

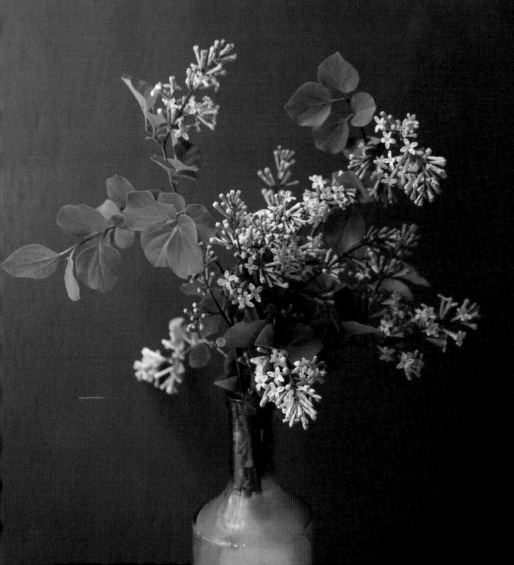

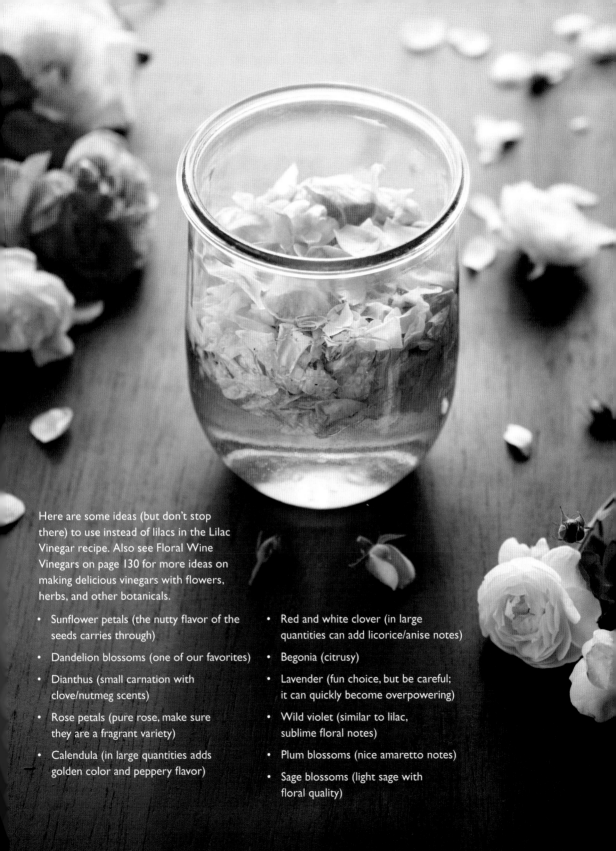

Here are some ideas (but don't stop there) to use instead of lilacs in the Lilac Vinegar recipe. Also see Floral Wine Vinegars on page 130 for more ideas on making delicious vinegars with flowers, herbs, and other botanicals.

- Sunflower petals (the nutty flavor of the seeds carries through)

- Dandelion blossoms (one of our favorites)

- Dianthus (small carnation with clove/nutmeg scents)

- Rose petals (pure rose, make sure they are a fragrant variety)

- Calendula (in large quantities adds golden color and peppery flavor)

- Red and white clover (in large quantities can add licorice/anise notes)

- Begonia (citrusy)

- Lavender (fun choice, but be careful; it can quickly become overpowering)

- Wild violet (similar to lilac, sublime floral notes)

- Plum blossoms (nice amaretto notes)

- Sage blossoms (light sage with floral quality)

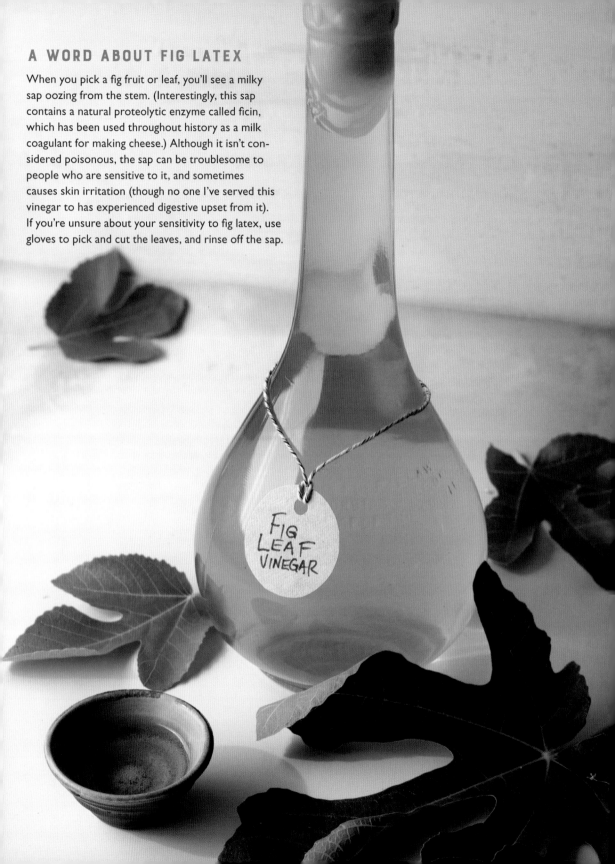

A WORD ABOUT FIG LATEX

When you pick a fig fruit or leaf, you'll see a milky
sap oozing from the stem. (Interestingly, this sap
contains a natural proteolytic enzyme called ficin,
which has been used throughout history as a milk
coagulant for making cheese.) Although it isn't considered poisonous, the sap can be troublesome to
people who are sensitive to it, and sometimes
causes skin irritation (though no one I've served this
vinegar to has experienced digestive upset from it).
If you're unsure about your sensitivity to fig latex, use
gloves to pick and cut the leaves, and rinse off the sap.

FIG
LEAF
VINEGAR

Fig Leaf Vinegar

THIS IS HANDS-DOWN one of my personal favorite vinegars. It's quick because it's made by the kitchen-counter Boerhaave method (page 94), in two half-gallon jars packed with fresh fig leaves from the common, fruit-producing fig (*Ficus carica*), not the houseplant. This gives it a unique flavor. How does one describe the flavor of fig leaves? Coconut notes come to mind, but it is much lighter than that; somehow there is a floral quality, too. This vinegar can be made with any fruit wine, but I think that cider or white wine yields the best results.

YIELD
1 gallon

4 cups (300 g) fresh fig leaves, or more as needed

1–2 cups (237–473 mL) raw, unpasteurized, unfiltered vinegar

¾ gallon (2.8 L) fermented hard cider, or 3 bottles white wine vinegar (2.25 L) diluted with 3 cups (710 mL) unchlorinated water

1. Let the leaves dry out for an hour or two, then cut them into 1- to 2-inch pieces with scissors. Divide the leaves to evenly fill a third of the way up in each of two sanitized half-gallon jars. Pour the vinegar over the leaves of one jar until they are submerged. Press the leaves down tightly. Let the leaves marinate for an hour or two. Pour off the vinegar into the second jar. Repeat the soaking time. Drain the remaining vinegar from the second jar, strain it, and bottle to store or use: It will also have some infused fig leaf flavor. Alternatively, you can put it in one of the jars and it will become part of the new vinegar.

2. Fill one jar to the top with the cider or diluted wine. This will give you the starting amount. Now pour about one-quarter of that into the second jar. You will have one jar that is three-quarters full and another that is one-quarter full.

3. Cover the jar with a basket-style coffee filter or a piece of unbleached cotton (butter muslin or tightly woven cheesecloth). Secure with a string, a rubber band, or a threaded metal canning band. This is to keep out fruit flies.

4. Place the jars in a spot that is warm (75° to 86°F/25° to 30°C; see page 71 for more specifics on temperature) and convenient, because you will be working with them daily.

5. The next day, pour the liquid from the nearly full jar into the other jar, leaving about one-quarter in the bottom of the first jar, exposing most of the filler material. This will move oxygen through the liquid and give the bacteria on the

recipe continues on next page

filler material time to "breathe." Do this once daily, or two to three times a day to speed the process.

6. In a few days, you will start to smell the distinctive vinegar aroma. Continue to transfer from jar to jar. Assuming a once-a-day transfer in an ambient home temperature, in 7 to 10 days you will have a young vinegar.

7. To make a finished vinegar, keep going. In 2 to 4 weeks, you should have a finished vinegar. You can take some off to bottle, or use it immediately and add new cider or wine to the jar; you will not need to dilute the wine this time for a continuous brew. Otherwise, bottle it all to use or age it and make another batch.

8. Use the leaves up to two more times. After the first round, the process will be faster because the leaves are fully inoculated. In fact, you will at some point see bits of mother forming on the leaves.

WINE VINEGAR

Sure, you can just leave a bottle out and oxidation will begin on its own. However, to make a delicious bottle of vinegar leaving less to chance, there are a few simple things to keep in mind. For example, adding a starter vinegar (with or without the MOV) helps make sure the acidity falls below pH 4.0 and encourages the ferment to happen faster. Once you have white wine mother and red wine mother cultures, you can make wine vinegar easily every time you want to.

Always check to see if the wine has sulfites. If it does, be sure to remove them (see page 43).

The other thing to be aware of is that most wine has an ABV that is too high for the vinegar bacteria to thrive in. (The wine gamut ranges from an impressive 5 to 23 percent ABV, with most falling in the 10 to 15 percent range.) If you have a wine that does not turn, it's likely because the alcohol level is too high (see page 41). The Universal Wine Vinegar recipe (page 129) is designed to work with wines in the average ABV range, by adding a third of the volume of wine in water.

Universal Wine Vinegar

THIS RECIPE WORKS with any type of wine—red, white, rosé, or a mix if you find yourself with many open bottles after a party. It's also a great way to use wines you don't like or ones that are corked. (This is a fault detected in bottled wine tainted by TCA, a compound that makes it taste more like wet dog than wine. The good news is that these wines will still make good vinegar.) Use this to make one batch, or keep the vinegar going by using some and adding more wine to the jar. Head to page 90 for more details on a continuous-brew method that can be done in a vinegar pot outfitted with a spigot.

**YIELD
about
1 quart**

1   bottle (750 mL) wine

½   teaspoon (2.5 mL) 3% hydrogen peroxide (if the wine contains sulfites)

1   cup (237 mL) unchlorinated water

½   cup (118 mL) raw, unfiltered, unpasteurized vinegar, or a vinegar mother

1. Pour the wine into a sanitized widemouthed jar. If the wine contains sulfites, stir in the hydrogen peroxide to neutralize them. Let sit for a minute. Stir in the water with a wooden spoon.

2. Pour in the raw vinegar. Stir well; a little oxygen is good for getting the process going.

3. Cover the jar with a piece of unbleached cotton (butter muslin or tightly woven cheesecloth), or a basket-style paper coffee filter. Secure with a string, a rubber band, or a threaded metal canning band. This is to keep out fruit flies.

4. Place on your counter or in another spot that is 75° to 86°F/25° to 30°C.

5. Check the vinegar in a month, when you should have nice acidity. However, it may take another month or two for the acidity to fully develop. Test the pH: It should be 4.0 or below.

6. Bottle half the vinegar and replace with the same amount of wine for another batch. Or bottle it all and store the mother for another batch or to share with a friend. Use immediately, or age to allow it to mellow and flavors to develop.

Variation:
Floral Wine Vinegars

AT TIMES, you may want to add delicate botanicals such as flower petals to give special essence and aroma to your wine vinegar. You have great leeway for how many blossoms to include. I generally use what I have, whether it's in my garden or what I can harvest sustainably. For example, I adore manzanita blossoms for cider flavoring, but these tiny flowers aren't abundant (though they are powerful; a mere quarter cup can flavor a whole gallon). However, I can pack a jar with calendula or rose petals, or begonia blossoms, because they are abundant. A good rule is to add a lightly packed cup of petals for each bottle of wine. If you're using delicately flavored flowers and you have a lot of them, feel free to use more. For floral vinegars, choose light wines like Riesling, Pinot Gris, Chardonnay, or Gewürztraminer.

YIELD
about 1 bottle
(750 mL)

1 bottle (750 mL) wine

1–2 cups lightly packed blossoms or petals, or florets picked from the stems, or more to taste

1. If the wine contains sulfites, follow steps 1 and 2 of Universal Wine Vinegar (page 129) for removing the sulfites and diluting with water.

2. Put the blossoms in a sanitized half-gallon jar. Use a wooden spoon to lightly crush the blossoms (the bruising will help release sugars and extract flavor).

3. Pour the prepared wine on the flowers. Continue with steps 3 through 6 of Universal Wine Vinegar.

HOW TO IDENTIFY A TRUE BALSAMIC

The process of making true, traditional balsamic vinegar is shrouded in evocative descriptions and near truths, so putting your finger on the exact method is difficult. This is just the way the makers of Modena like it. (But I'm jumping ahead a bit.)

IS IT REALLY BALSAMIC?

First, it's important to understand that a bottle of balsamic is not necessarily a bottle of balsamic. The vinegar that most of us think of when we hear the word *balsamic* is the industrially produced Aceto Balsamico di Modena (Balsamic of Modena), which was introduced in the 1960s. The process of making true, traditional balsamic takes years and involves a slow relay of aging in ever-smaller barrels made of different types of wood. At the writing of this book, there were only 67 makers of Aceto Balsamico Tradizionale whose product received the Denominazione di Origine Protetta (DOP) status. Three of these makers control 80 percent of this rare vinegar, and only one is located outside Italy (see page 112). Aceto Balsamico Tradizionale itself accounts for a mere 0.01 percent of the market.

READ THE LABEL (AND THE PRICE TAG)

Most people don't realize they've never tasted real balsamic. Blame the confusing labels; there are many tricky ways to make a product sound like the real thing. For example, one label promises a pleasant dark, thick "Modena District" made with just wine vinegar and grape must; declares it is a "Cherry Wood Aged Balsamic Grand Reserve Vinegar"; brandishes 25 stars; and repeats the word *aged* three times in just 19 words. When I initially saw the number 25, I assumed (incorrectly, it turned out)

25 years of aging. Brilliant marketing! The retail price of this product was a dead giveaway, though. A bottle of true balsamic is easily $60 or more an ounce—an understandable price, when you realize that each bottle of true balsamic contains the equivalent of many reduced bottles of wine. And true balsamic contains only grapes—no sugar or caramel coloring.

EXAMINE THE DENSITY

Aceto Balsamico Tradizionale (traditional balsamic vinegar, or TBV) is dense due to the slow evaporation over years. In fact, the product is considered a *condimento* (condiment), and is not officially an *aceto* (vinegar) until its twelfth birthday, when aging of a TBV begins to count. *Extra vecchio* means the vinegar has matured for at least 25 years. A gallon of this aged vinegar can weigh anywhere from 23 to 26 pounds (in contrast, water weighs 8 pounds per gallon).

When you go to a restaurant and your beautifully plated food comes with artfully drizzled syrupy balsamic, it is most likely a Balsamic of Modena that has been reduced with heat (as is the recipe on page 121). In most restaurants, it isn't financially feasible to use TBV, and to the untrained eye and palate, Balsamic of Modena is an easy substitute. If the vinegar is viscous and gummy, it's a cooked reduction. The flavor will also be syrupy, and the acidity will be faint, if even present at all. If it is thick (dense, not viscous), very dark, yet clear and smooth, and sweet and acidic, then you may be enjoying Aceto Balsamico Tradizionale.

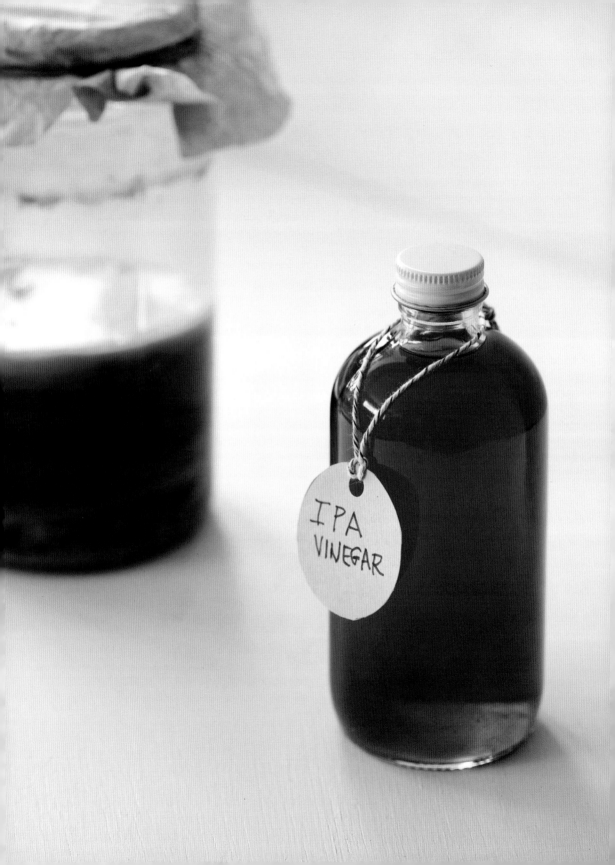

Beer Vinegar

THE BEAUTIFUL THING ABOUT beer vinegar is that the ABV is right where you need it to be. Technically, you can just pour the beer into an open container and watch it go flat. That said, this vinegar can been hit or miss, depending on which microbes move in first, and some beers are more susceptible to surface yeast than others. To avoid unwanted yeast, add a starter vinegar. The starter can be any raw vinegar; after that, you'll have beer-centric MOVs. For example, I have a deep, dark porter vinegar and a hoppy vinegar from a hop-heavy IPA. (There is a lot of online chatter that you can't make vinegar with a hoppy beer, which isn't true. I believe this misconception stems from the fact that hops have antimicrobial and preservative qualities.) Ultimately, use whatever beer you like—the diversity is almost dizzying. The one parameter is to make sure your alcohol level isn't higher than 9 percent, or you'll need to add a little unchlorinated water to dilute it.

**YIELD
about
1½ quarts**

3 pints (1.4 L) beer from three 16-ounce cans or four 12-ounce cans

1¼ cups (296 mL) raw, unfiltered, unpasteurized vinegar, with the mother, if available

1. Pour the beer into a sanitized half-gallon jar. Allow it to settle and go flat.

2. When the carbonation is gone, pour in the vinegar with the mother, if available. Stir well with a wooden spoon; a little oxygen is always good for getting the process going.

3. Cover the jar with a piece of unbleached cotton (butter muslin or tightly woven cheesecloth), or a basket-style paper coffee filter. Secure with a string, a rubber band, or a threaded metal canning band. This is to keep out fruit flies.

4. Place on your counter or in another spot that is 75° to 86°F/25° to 30°C.

5. Check the vinegar in a month, when you should have nice acidity. However, it may take another month or two to fully develop. Test the pH: It should be 4.0 or below.

6. Bottle half the vinegar and replace with the same amount of beer for another batch. Or bottle it all and store the mother for next time or share with a friend.

7. Use immediately, or age to allow it to mellow and flavors to develop.

Doburoku-Method Rice Wine Vinegar

DOBUROKU IS THE CLOUDY farmhouse-style sake, also known as rice wine. If you want to make doburoku starting from rice or any other grain, you will start by making an amazake; follow the instructions on page 87. Consider this recipe the final step. If you want to make rice wine vinegar but don't want to go to the trouble of making doburoku first, you can substitute a well-made purchased sake in this recipe. These rustic grain wines are high in alcohol and must be thinned with water. You can also refer to this recipe when you're making any vinegar that comes from an amazake process (see page 87).

As with all vinegars, you can seed it with unpasteurized vinegar or your own raw vinegar and mother, or you can wait for the acetic bacteria in the air to move in. If you choose to go with a wild fermentation, it is important to stir the young vinegar every day. This will help accelerate the process and will keep surface yeasts from forming.

YIELD
about 1 gallon

1 recipe doburoku (see page 219) or about 3½ quarts (3.3 L) purchased sake

6 cups (1.4 L) water

2 cups (473 mL) raw, unfiltered, unpasteurized vinegar, with the mother, if available

1. Combine the doburoku and water in a sanitized crock or other open fermentation vessel. Add the vinegar and stir with a wooden spoon.

2. Cover the crock with muslin or any cloth that will allow air circulation. Secure the cloth around the rim with a string or rubber band.

3. Ferment in a warm spot, preferably 75° to 86°F/25° to 30°C, stirring daily for the first 2 weeks. If you are using a mother, place it on top of the liquid now. If not, continue to stir as needed, if you see surface yeasts developing during the continued fermentation for 6 weeks to 2 months. The vinegar is finished when it tastes right to you. At this point, test the pH: It should be 4.0 or below.

4. Bottle the vinegar—either as is, or strained and filtered—in an airtight bottle. Use immediately, or age to allow it to mellow and develop flavors.

Gin-egar

I RARELY HAVE A COCKTAIL, but when I do it is a gin and tonic and I silently raise my glass to my Great Aunt Eleanor, who loved G&Ts and taught me never to grow up. My home state also has some amazing small distillers making fantastic gin, so that's another good reason to make it my go-to spirit. That said, don't feel like you need to buy top-shelf liquor for this vinegar. Quality inputs are always important, but the cheaper stuff works well. Because the base is distilled, it lacks the nutrients necessary for the bacteria to be in top form. The small amount of beer in this recipe gives them what they need. If you can find an unpasteurized white wine vinegar, or have light-colored raw vinegars, use those as your starter (I used corncob vinegar; see page 184). This will retain the clarity and mood of the gin. However, ACV will still create a fine product.

This recipe works with any type of 80 proof alcohol—rum, bourbon, mezcal, brandy, schnapps, tequila, pisco—so choose your favorite. These feel like daring flavors that can be used in cooking, but also are wonderful as part of cocktails or mocktails. Think about what you're looking for in the final product; for example, a smoky mescal will give you some lingering smoky notes.

YIELD
about
2½ quarts

1 fifth (750 mL) gin

2 quarts (1.9 L) room-temperature unchlorinated water

2 tablespoons beer; use a lighter beer if you want a clearer color

2 cups (473 mL) raw, unfiltered, unpasteurized vinegar, or a vinegar mother

1. Pour the gin, water, beer, and vinegar starter into a sanitized widemouthed gallon jar.

2. Stir well; a little oxygen is good for getting the process going.

3. Cover the jar with a piece of unbleached cotton (butter muslin or tightly woven cheesecloth), or a basket-style paper coffee filter. Secure with a string, a rubber band, or a threaded metal canning band. This is to keep out fruit flies.

4. Place on your counter or in another spot that is 75° to 86°F/25° to 30°C.

5. Check the vinegar in a month, when you should have nice acidity. However, it may take another month or two for the acidity to fully develop. Test the pH: It should be 4.0 or below.

6. Bottle the vinegar in an airtight bottle. Use immediately, or age to allow it to mellow and develop flavors.

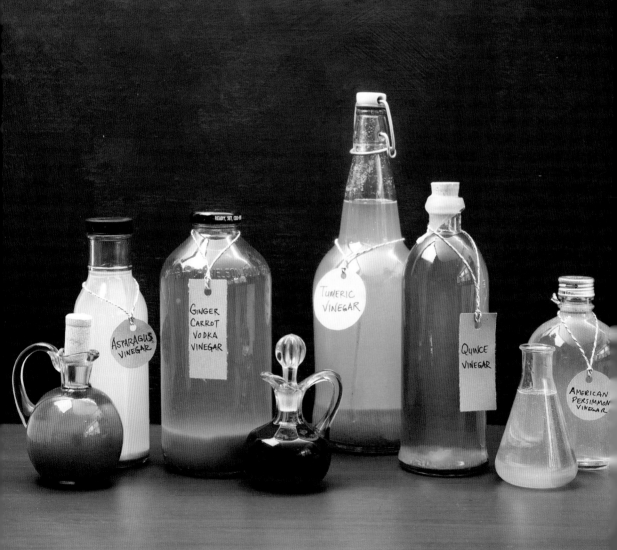

ASPARAGUS VINEGAR

GINGER CARROT VODKA VINEGAR

TUMERIC VINEGAR

QUINCE VINEGAR

AMERICAN PERSIMMON VINEGAR

READY, SET, GU-M

CHAPTER 6

VINEGARS FROM FRESH FRUITS AND VEGGIES

MAKING VINEGAR FROM FRUIT is a no-brainer. Wild yeast and acetic bacteria are already present on the fruit, so if you mash fruit and wait long enough, you'll have vinegar. (See the recipe for Japanese Persimmon Vinegar on page 150.) It's no wonder that fruit vinegars are found in ancient cultures across the globe. People ate according to the seasons; fruit came in and rotted very quickly without refrigeration. Vinegar not only provided a way to preserve the nutrients in the fruit at hand but also helped preserve other fruits and foods.

VINEGAR FROM WHAT'S AT HAND

In Europe, and then the New World, apples and grapes gave us cider and wine first, then vinegar. Throughout the Middle East, vinegar was made with dates. In the Jeongeup-si and Jeollabuk-do regions of southwestern Korea, a vinegar was made with small native persimmons. In fact, a Korean agriculture manual from 1827 lists 42 different vinegar recipes using not just persimmons but rice, barley, jujubes, peaches, honey, and tangerines.

Regional resources led to regional vinegars and distinctive styles of making all over the world. In the Philippines, fresh coconut sap, called *tubâ*, became coconut vinegar. In Mexico, pineapple vinegar was made from the fruit's peels. Over time, the Modena region of Italy produced a fruit vinegar that uniquely developed there—balsamic.

In this chapter, you'll find recipes that are built off that notion of seasonal abundance. When you have extra, you can preserve the antioxidants and flavors in a shelf-stable manner to be enjoyed throughout the year. If you have fruit and vegetables that you don't see here, which you undoubtedly will, remember that any country/fruit wine recipe will get you started. After a couple of weeks of fermentation, you can add about a half cup of unpasteurized vinegar for every half gallon of wine you make.

LET'S TALK ABOUT FERMENTABLE SUGARS

There are two types of sugar in our fruits and vegetables—simple sugars and complex sugars. Complex sugars are also known as starch and are often in the form of polysaccharides (complex carbohydrates). We're after simple sugars when we make vinegar, because they are the fermentable sugars. They are like candy; these sugars are immediately available for the microbes. Fruit starts with more starch, and as ripening accelerates, the sugars become more available. The starch disappears from the center of the fruit, moves outward, and loses a bit of moisture, effectively condensing the sugars that remain. When you're making vinegar, it's best to let your berries and fruits overripen, to get the most fermentable sugar. The mealy apple and the brown banana that get passed up in the fruit bowl are perfect for this job.

Vegetables are the opposite. When they're growing, they generate simple sugars, such as glucose and fructose, through photosynthesis. When you make vinegar from vegetables, use fresh, in-season produce, because the sugar that feeds the microbes slowly dries out or converts to starch, becoming less available the longer it's stored after harvest. I have seen cabbages that wouldn't ferment because they were too dry. In this case, the dehydration doesn't condense the sugars in a positive way. When root vegetables are freshly dug from the ground, they're juicy and full of simple sugar. When in long-term storage, the root is waiting to grow again, and sugars travel through the root and metabolize into starch. This makes the fermentation less active, and in some cases, it will require more simple sugar added to get a strong alcohol.

Blackberry/Raspberry Vinegar

THIS RECIPE MAKES A BEAUTIFUL deep purple-red vinegar with a nice acidity and berry notes. Raspberry is lighter in both acidity and color than blackberry. Vinegar made from any type of berry will brighten up the color and flavor of a vinaigrette. Feel free to use blackberries (or any of their cousins: marionberries, boysenberries, loganberries, olallieberries, and so on), raspberries, or a combination of the two. This is a simultaneous ferment, meaning the yeast and the bacteria starter are added at the same time.

YIELD
1½ quarts

1 pound (450 g) mashed berries, can be overripe

¾ cup (155 g) sugar, any kind

2 quarts (1.9 L) unchlorinated water, just off the boil

½ teaspoon (1 g) wine yeast, hydrated in ¼ cup (59 mL) unchlorinated water, warmed to 104°F/40°C; or ½ cup (118 mL) room-temperature wild yeast starter (page 53)

½ cup (118 mL) raw, unfiltered, unpasteurized vinegar, or a vinegar mother

1. Combine the fruit and sugar in a sanitized half-gallon jar. Add the just-boiled water and fill within 2 to 3 inches of the top of the jar. Cool to room temperature.

2. Add the hydrated yeast or the wild yeast starter to the jar. Stir well.

3. Add the raw vinegar. Stir well with a wooden spoon. Unlike with most ferments, you want to get oxygen in the mix. However, make sure the mashed berries stay submerged; otherwise they can become a host for undesirable opportunistic bacteria.

4. Cover the jar with a piece of unbleached cotton (butter muslin or tightly woven cheesecloth), or a basket-style paper coffee filter. Secure with a string, a rubber band, or a threaded metal canning band. This is to keep out fruit flies.

5. Place on your counter or in another spot that is 75° to 86°F/25° to 30°C.

6. Stir with a wooden spoon once a day for the first 5 or 6 days. After that, stir now and then, if you remember. You may see bubbles: That is good.

recipe continues on next page

7. The ferment will begin to slow down in about 2 weeks. Then it's time to take out the scraps. When you remove the cover, you may see a film developing on top. It is the beginning of the vinegar mother. Remove and set it aside while you're straining out the fruit solids.

8. Transfer the strained almost-vinegar (and the vinegar mother, if you have one) to a clean jar and cover again.

9. Check the vinegar in a month, when you should have nice acidity. However, it may take another month or two to fully develop. Test the pH: It should be 4.0 or below.

10. Bottle the finished vinegar, saving the mother for another batch or sharing with a friend.

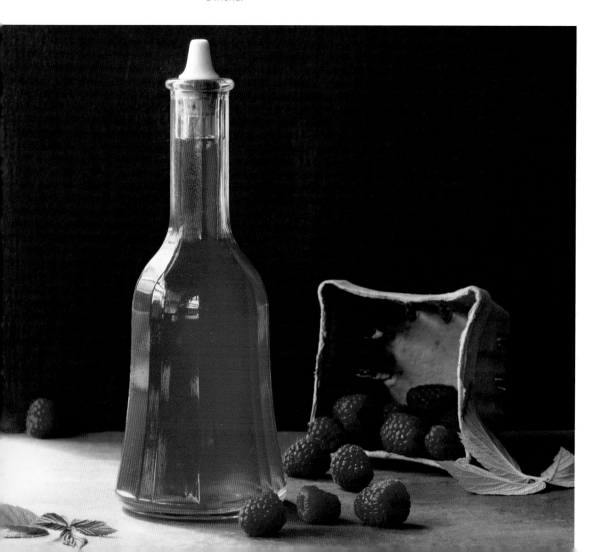

Carrot-Ginger Vinegar

THE BRIGHT ORANGE color of this vinegar is reason enough to make it—the flavor is the other reason. It is a bright and cheery light vinegar that is at the same time grounded by the hint of spicy ginger. It's important to note that the fine carrot pulp, which provides the color, settles to the bottom on the shelf. Shake upon use. For a smoother vinegar, you can strain out the bulk of the larger pulp, as the recipe indicates; the extra texture is slightly gritty. After making it a number of times strained, I realized that, since I use it mostly on salad anyway, the pulp isn't an issue.

This is an example of a recipe that skips the first yeast fermentation and uses ethanol, in the form of vodka, to feed the acetic bacteria. Feel free to play around with this technique with other juiced vegetables. You'll need a juicer for this recipe.

YIELD
1½ quarts

4.4 pounds (2 kg) carrots

1 2- to 3-inch piece (45 g) fresh ginger

1 cup + 2 tablespoons (245 mL) vodka

1 cup (237 mL) raw, unfiltered, unpasteurized vinegar, or a vinegar mother

1. Scrub and juice the carrots and the ginger. You will end up with almost a quart (0.9 L) of juice. (Make carrot bread with the pulp.)

2. Put the juice in a sanitized half-gallon jar. Add the vodka and vinegar. Stir well with a wooden spoon. Unlike with most ferments, you want to get some oxygen in the mix.

3. Cover the jar with a piece of unbleached cotton (butter muslin or tightly woven cheesecloth), or a basket-style paper coffee filter. Secure with a string, a rubber band, or a threaded metal canning band. This is to keep out fruit flies.

4. Place on your counter or in a spot that is 75° to 86°F/25° to 30°C.

5. Stir once a day for the first 5 or 6 days, or longer. The fine pulp will continue to separate in the jar, so continued stirring is good to keep the oxygen throughout the mix. Check the vinegar in a month, when you should have nice acidity. However, it may take another month or two to fully develop, especially if your environment is cooler.

6. Pour the mixture through a fine-mesh sieve to strain out most of the pulp. Save the pulp to use anywhere you want some bright orange acidity; it is delicious. Bottle the finished vinegar, saving the mother for another batch or sharing with a friend.

7. Use immediately, or age to allow it to mellow and develop flavors. The color will continue to separate as it sits, so shake each time you use the vinegar.

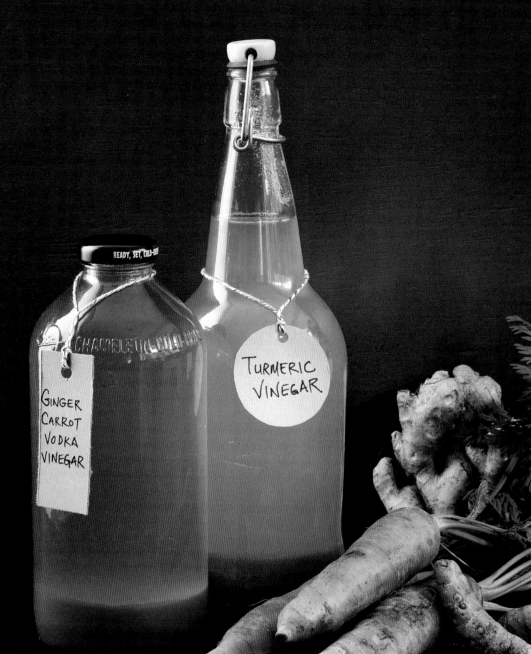

GINGER
CARROT
VODKA
VINEGAR

TURMERIC
VINEGAR

READY, SET, COLD-BRE

Turmeric Vinegar

TURMERIC VINEGAR WILL light up your world. I use this for vinegar drinks—this vinegar in a little sparkling water with some ice is a refreshing beverage. The earthiness of turmeric comes through beautifully. I also use this for making mustard and brightening up a curry. If you're a fan of ginger, this same recipe can be made with fresh ginger instead of turmeric. Use any type of sugar. I generally use raw cane sugar, but feel free to use white sugar because it works well and is so much more affordable. As an aside, I have never seen a mother form on this vinegar or the fresh ginger variation.

YIELD
about 2 quarts

⅔ cup (200 g) fresh turmeric root, grated

1 cup (200 g) sugar, any kind

6 cups (1.4 L) unchlorinated water, warmed to 85°F/29°C

½ teaspoon (1 g) wine yeast hydrated in ¼ cup (59 mL) unchlorinated water, warmed to 104°F/40°C; or ½ cup (118 mL) room-temperature wild yeast starter (page 53)

1¼ cups (296 mL) raw, unfiltered, unpasteurized vinegar, or a vinegar mother

1. Put the turmeric in a sanitized half-gallon jar. Stir in the sugar and 6 cups water.

2. Add the hydrated yeast or wild yeast starter to the jar. Stir well with a wooden spoon.

3. Cover the jar with a piece of unbleached cotton (butter muslin or tightly woven cheesecloth), or a basket-style paper coffee filter. Secure with a string, a rubber band, or a threaded metal canning band. This is to keep out fruit flies.

4. Place on your counter. You may see bubbles: That is good. In my experience, turmeric takes a little longer than other ferments to get boozy.

5. After 7 to 10 days, add the raw vinegar. Stir again and replace the cover. Set the jar in a spot that is ideally 75° to 86°F/25° to 30°C. Stir occasionally to kick up the turmeric mash and oxygenate.

recipe continues on next page

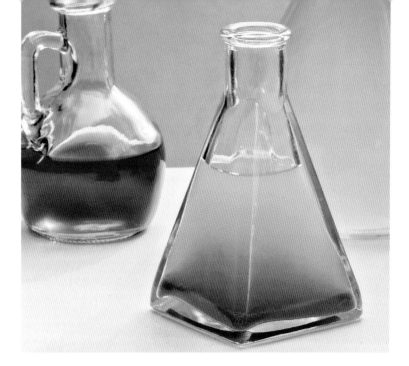

6. Check the vinegar in a month, when you should have nice acidity. However, it may take another month or two to fully develop, especially if your environment is cooler. In my experience with this vinegar, there is no mother development. Check the pH: It should be 4.0 or below.

7. When the vinegar has reached the desired acidity, either pour the mixture through a fine-mesh sieve to strain out most of the pulp, or keep the turmeric in and shake the vinegar before use. (If you strain, save the pulp to use in any dishes where you want some bright anti-inflammatory acidity.)

8. Bottle the finished vinegar. Use immediately (shaking before each use), or age to allow it to mellow and develop flavors. The color will continue to separate as it sits.

FRUITLESS VINEGARS

Commercial fruit and vegetable vinegars may or may not have been made from the fruit or vegetable that's on the label. Often, no fruit or vegetable was ever fermented in the process. Many artisanal berry vinegars are made by infusing berries into a commercial white vinegar; the better ones use white wine vinegars. Commercial vinegars don't even infuse whole fruits or vegetables; instead, they mix fruit or vegetable juices with distilled white vinegar. You will notice this if you start looking carefully at the labels of gourmet vinegars. You will see fruit flavors and essences added to more common vinegars made from apples, grapes, grains, or unidentified white vinegar sources.

Hibiscus Vinegar

NATURALLY ACIDIC AND FRUITY, hibiscus is a wonderful choice for a beautiful, unique vinegar. It is a fantastic drinking vinegar—partly due to the color. This recipe uses dried hibiscus flowers that yield a beautiful deep red vinegar. You will find the flowers, whole or in pieces, in bulk sections of natural foods stores or sold as tea at import markets (and labeled as hibiscus or sorrel, an unrelated plant).

You can also use this as a base recipe for other herbal tisanes or botanical flavors that you want to capture in vinegar. Simply substitute other aromatics, singly or as a mix of a few, in place of the hibiscus. For example, one time I made a pot of mango Ceylon tea that we forgot to drink. I decided to process it as vinegar according to this recipe, and it was fantastic. Someday I intend to do the same with coffee. Another variation is to use fresh herbal preparations. For example, substitute 10 cups lightly packed fresh rose petals for the dried hibiscus to create rose vinegar.

YIELD
about 1 gallon

1 cup (60 g) dried hibiscus flowers

10 raisins

4½ cups (905 g) turbinado sugar

3½ quarts (3.3 L) unchlorinated water

½ teaspoon (1 g) wine yeast hydrated in ¼ cup (59 ml) unchlorinated water, warmed to 104°F/40°C; or ½ cup (118 mL) room-temperature wild yeast starter (page 53)

Juice of 1 lemon

1 cup (237 mL) raw, unfiltered, unpasteurized vinegar, or a vinegar mother

MAYBE YOU'RE WONDERING: WHY THE RAISINS? They give the yeast some extra nutrition. From the yeast's perspective, teas and tisanes are akin to sugar water. On its own, sugar water isn't quite enough for yeasts to thrive on.

1. Sanitize a gallon jar, keeping it slightly warm to avoid cracking when introducing hot materials later.

2. Combine the flowers and raisins in the warm jar. Alternatively, put the flowers and raisins in a winemaking straining bag and set that in the jar.

3. Combine the sugar and water in a stockpot. Bring to a boil, stirring until the sugar is completely dissolved.

4. Pour the boiling sugar water into the jar. Cover with a cloth or the jar's lid (not fully secured) and let steep for 24 hours.

recipe continues on next page

5. Remove the flowers and strain the liquid through cheesecloth, or pull out the straining bag, returning the liquid to the same jar. Squeeze the fabric to extract as much of flavorful juice as possible. Make sure this "tea" is room temperature.

6. Add the hydrated yeast or the wild yeast starter to the jar. Stir well with a wooden spoon.

7. Cover the jar with a piece of unbleached cotton (butter muslin or tightly woven cheesecloth), or a basket-style paper coffee filter. Secure with a string, a rubber band, or a threaded metal canning band. This is to keep out fruit flies. Keep at room temperature.

8. You may see bubbles: That is good. Stir with a wooden spoon now and then, if you remember. The ferment will begin to slow down in about 2 weeks.

9. When the fermentation has slowed, add the vinegar, and stir. Replace the cover and set the jar on your counter or in another spot that is 75° to 86°F/25° to 30°C. Stir occasionally to oxygenate. When you remove the cover, you may see a film developing on top. It is the beginning of the vinegar mother.

10. Check the vinegar in another month, when you should have nice acidity. However, it may take another month or two to fully develop, especially if your environment is cooler.

11. Bottle the finished vinegar, saving the mother for another batch or sharing with a friend. Use immediately, or age to allow it to mellow and develop flavors.

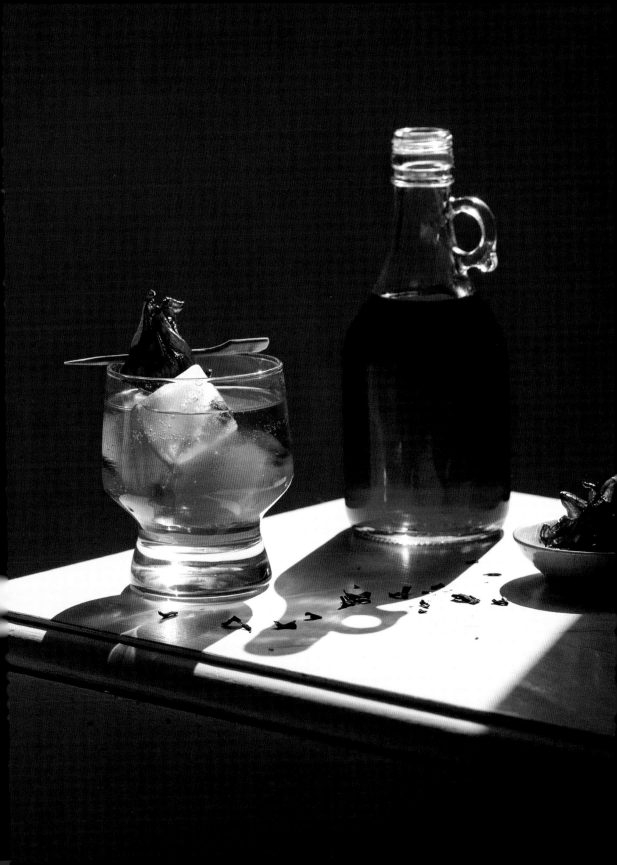

Wild American Persimmon Vinegar

KOREA HAS A LONG HISTORY with persimmon vinegar made from the small, native Meoski persimmons that are both sweet and tannic. According to the Slow Food Foundation for Biodiversity, this traditional vinegar was a staple made in most Korean households yet now is in danger of being lost. The Slow Food website describes the process of harvesting and drying the fruits and fermenting them in a raw alcohol, usually rice wine makgeolli. The wine takes on the persimmon fermentation, and when finished, the family's vinegar mother is added.

My variation is local to my valley and uses the native American persimmon in our homemade cider. I don't dry the persimmons but ferment them in the cider and turn this into vinegar. It is lovely. Use cider or sake for this recipe.

YIELD
about 1 quart

1 pound (454 g) American persimmons

1 quart (0.9 L) hard cider, or 3 cups (710 mL) rice wine diluted with
    1 cup (237 mL) unchlorinated water

1. Set the persimmons in a sanitized widemouthed half-gallon jar. Crush them lightly.

2. Pour the cider over the fruit. Stir well with a wooden spoon. Unlike with most ferments, you want to get some oxygen in the mix. However, make sure that the persimmons stay submerged. Otherwise they can become a host for undesirable opportunistic bacteria.

3. Cover the jar with a piece of unbleached cotton (butter muslin or tightly woven cheesecloth), or a basket-style paper coffee filter. Secure with a string, a rubber band, or a threaded metal canning band. This is to keep out fruit flies.

4. Place on your counter or in another spot that is 75° to 86°F/25° to 30°C.

5. Stir once a day for the first 5 or 6 days. After that, stir now and then, if you remember. You may see bubbles: That is good.

6. The ferment will slow down in about 2 weeks. Then it is time to strain out the persimmon mash. When you remove the cover, you may see a film developing on top. It is the beginning of the vinegar mother. Remove and set it aside. Line a strainer with a piece of butter muslin or fine-mesh cheesecloth and strain the mixture into a new sanitized jar. Press on the fruit and squeeze the cloth to get every last tasty drop out. Cover the jar.

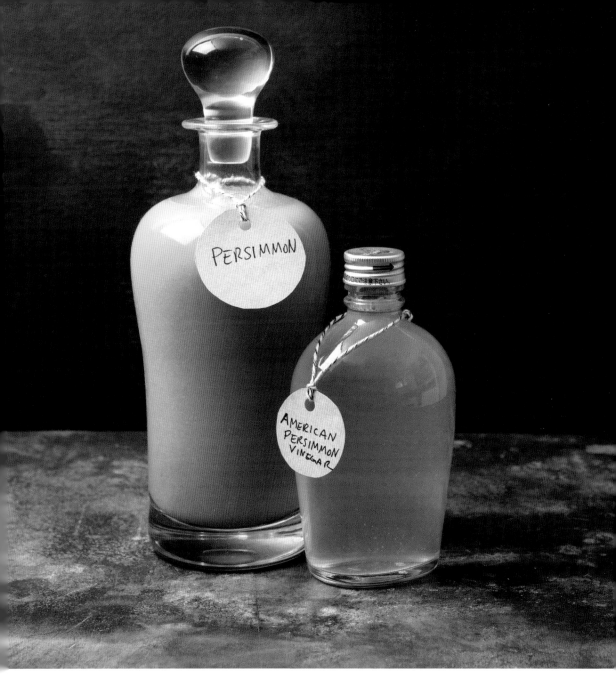

7. Check the vinegar in a month, when you should have nice acidity. However, it may take another month or two to fully develop, especially if your environment is cooler.

8. Bottle the finished vinegar, saving the mother for another batch or sharing with a friend. Use immediately, or age to allow it to mellow and develop flavors.

Japanese Persimmon Vinegar

THIS METHOD COMES directly from the wonderful book *Preserving the Japanese Way* by Nancy Singleton Hachisu. Use any type of persimmons, or a mix of varieties. You can use any quantity, but I found that it is good to have at least three pounds or more of fruit—partly because of the time involved to the amount gained, but also because, in my experience, with less than three pounds the project lacks enough mass to keep the fermenting fruit from going off.

YIELD
about 1½ quarts

3 pounds (1.3 kg) persimmons

¼ cup (59 mL) persimmon vinegar (optional)

1. Stuff the persimmons into a sanitized widemouthed gallon jar or crock, leaving 2 inches of headspace below the neck. Press with a tamper as you insert them into the jar to crush the fruit and push out air pockets.

2. If you have persimmon vinegar from a previous batch, stir it in now.

3. Cover the jar with a piece of unbleached cotton (butter muslin or tightly woven cheesecloth), or a basket-style paper coffee filter. Secure with a string, a rubber band, or a threaded metal canning band. This is to keep out fruit flies.

4. Set your vessel in a warm (75° to 86°F/25° to 30°C), visible spot so that you won't forget it. Nancy suggests a sunny location. You will need to stir it often for the first few weeks to build flavor and work out air pockets that if left too long can develop mold. I suggest stirring every day, because then you can build it into your routine. (Drink your coffee, stir your mushy persimmon baby . . .)

5. The mixture will soften, then turn effervescent. After the initial fermentation calms down, let the batch rest. Wait about 3 months before straining.

6. To strain, use a food mill if you have one. If not, line a strainer with a piece of butter muslin or fine-mesh cheesecloth and strain the mixture into a new sanitized jar. Press on the fruit and squeeze the cloth to get every last tasty drop out.

7. Bottle the finished vinegar. Use immediately, or age to allow it to mellow and develop flavors. The next time, you can use some of this as a starter, and it will help the new batch move a little bit faster.

VINEGAR STUDY:
TAMARIND VINEGAR

I love the flavor of tamarind and use it when I can, so I decided to try making vinegar from the fruit. It was a tasty vinegar, but the final product tasted very much like ACV—so much so that it wasn't worth my time to make it, given that apples are local and tamarind is not. Here are the notes from my experiment; it's not a tested recipe. If you live in an area where tamarind is abundant and apples are not, you can make tamarind vinegar in the following manner.

Soak 11 ounces (325 g) of peeled fruit in 2 quarts (1.9 L) of unchlorinated water, just off the boil, for 48 hours. Pull the pits from the pulp. If you have a hydrometer and are curious, take a specific gravity reading of the liquid. If not, add 1 cup (250 g) of sugar. When I did the reading, was 1.030, which is a little low for a 4 to 6 percent vinegar, and that's why I added the cup of sugar to bring it to 1.070. To this I added ½ teaspoon of wine yeast and let the fermentation begin in a widemouthed jar with a coffee-filter topper. After the first week, I strained out the extra pulp and added 1 cup (237 mL) of raw ACV. After 6 weeks, the mother formed, and the vinegar was well under way. I bottled it at 2 months.

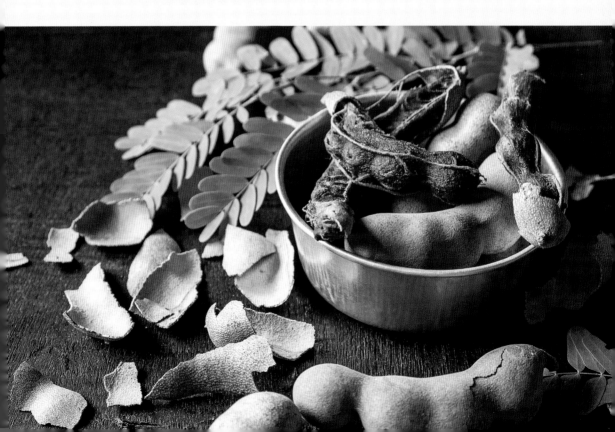

Chocolate Vinegar

DURING THE WRITING of this book, I was chocolate nib rich, thanks to my dear friend and fellow food writer, Karen Solomon. I was experimenting with growing koji on nibs, so I had some cocoa-scented soaking water that smelled too delicious to dump. Since I was in an all-things-can-be-vinegar state of mind, you know what happened next.

A few days into the alcohol fermentation, the product was unstable but amazing. Sweetness still held the bitterness in check—yum! That stage was brief. The yeast kept consuming sugar, and soon there was a very bitter alcohol that became a very bitter vinegar. I had multiple batches, in order to test different ratios; they were all bitter. I didn't throw the vinegars away; they smelled too good! Instead, they aged in the bottle. I would taste them once in a while and think, "Yuck." (This from someone who loves 90 percent cacao or higher bitter dark chocolate.)

After six months, the flavors turned. Suddenly this vinegar was an example of how esters develop and flavors increase over time. The vinegar became delicious. The chocolate nose was stronger, the bitterness took a back seat, and the acidity mellowed. I can't wait to see what it does after a year.

YIELD
1½ quarts

3 cups (342 g) cacao nibs

5⅓ cups (1262 mL) room-temperature, unchlorinated water

½ teaspoon (1 g) wine yeast hydrated in ¼ cup (59 mL) unchlorinated water, warmed to 104°F/40°C; or ½ cup (118 mL) room-temperature wild yeast starter (page 53)

1¼ cups (296 mL) raw, unfiltered, unpasteurized vinegar, or a vinegar mother

¾ cup (170 g) sugar, any kind

1. Place the nibs in a nonreactive saucepan with the water. Warm gently, and keep at 140°F/60°C for 1 hour. Keep a lid on the pan to avoid too much evaporation. Alternatively, vacuum-seal the nibs and water in a sealed plastic bag and keep at 140°F/60°C for 1 hour in a sous vide water bath or in a pot of hot water.

2. Strain the nibs from the chocolate water. (Use the nibs for making koji—see the instructions on page 277—toast and add to granola, or bake with them. They still have plenty of flavor.)

3. Transfer the chocolate water to a sanitized half-gallon jar. Stir in the sugar.

4. Add the hydrated yeast or the wild yeast starter to the jar. Stir well with a wooden spoon.

5. Cover the jar with a piece of unbleached cotton (butter muslin or tightly woven cheesecloth), or a basket-style paper coffee filter. Secure with a string, a rubber band, or a threaded metal canning band. This is to keep out fruit flies. Keep at room temperature.

6. After 7 days, add the vinegar and stir. Replace the cover and place the jar on your counter or in another spot that is 75° to 86°F/25° to 30°C.

7. Check the vinegar in a month, when you should have nice acidity. However, it will be quite bitter at this point and not worth trying to use. Instead, bottle the vinegar and age for at least 6 months to allow it to mellow and develop flavors.

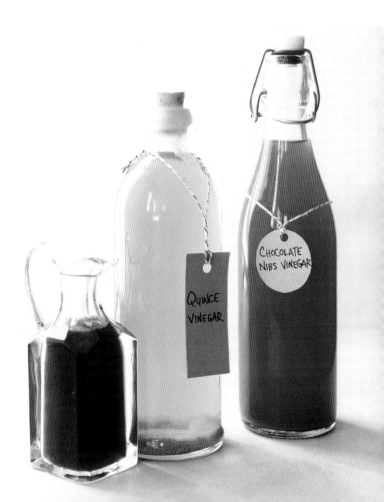

Quince Vinegar

THIS IS ONE OF MY FAVORITE vinegars but I am not going to lie: Preparing quince (*Cydonia oblonga*) is not easy. It is a rock-hard fruit that needs to be peeled, cored, and grated. This vinegar is worth the effort, though I admit to not thinking so (insert grumbly thought bubble) when I am grating the fruit. The flavor of quince in the vinegar is immediately recognizable. Quince vinegar will surprise you with its slightly sweet, tropical mood.

What's quince? you ask. A misshapen pear with a bad haircut? This fruit is in the same family as apples, pears, hawthorn berries, and roses. It is slightly fuzzy, like a peach, but the fuzz can be rubbed off easily as it ripens. In general, quinces are not eaten raw, as they are quite astringent and don't soften and ripen right away— although I received a sweet note from a reader in South Africa assuring me that he's eaten them raw his whole life and that the "astringent taste goes very well with salt." I will try that next season.

YIELD
about 1 gallon

3 pounds (1.36 kg) overripe quinces

3½ quarts (3.3 L) unchlorinated water

2½ cups (565 g) sugar, any kind

Juice of 1 lemon

½ teaspoon (1 g) wine yeast hydrated in ¼ cup (59 ml) unchlorinated water, warmed to 104°F/40°C; or ½ cup (118 mL) room-temperature wild yeast starter (page 53)

1 cup (237 mL) raw, unfiltered, unpasteurized vinegar, or a vinegar mother

1. Be sure the quinces have overripened, which will look less like the softening you are used to with other fruit. The fuzzy exterior will rub off easily, and the quinces will almost feel a little greasy. You want them developed as much as possible but not darkened or brown. Scrub clean.

2. Grate the fruit on a box grater or with a grating attachment on a food processor. (Roughly chopping and pulsing the fruit in the food processor doesn't work well.)

3. Combine the grated quinces, water, sugar, and lemon juice in a large nonreactive pot. Bring to a simmer over medium heat, then reduce the heat to low and simmer until the fruit is soft and cooked. As it cooks, it turns a pretty peachy pink color.

4. Transfer the mixture into a lidded plastic food-safe bucket, Cambro container, or another sanitized vessel. Let cool to around 100°F/38°C.

5. When the quince mixture has cooled, add the hydrated yeast or wild starter. Stir with a wooden spoon until well mixed. Cover the container with the lid. Let the mixture sit for 48 hours, stirring twice a day and replacing the lid. Unlike with most ferments, you want to get oxygen in the mix. However, make sure the fruit scraps stay submerged, otherwise they can become a host for undesirable opportunistic bacteria.

6. After 2 days, strain out the quince, either by pressing it through cheesecloth or a using a vegetable food mill. (Save the pulp to make a quince butter, or bake with it.)

7. Place the strained mixture in a sanitized gallon jar. It should be beginning to actively ferment. Cover the jar with a piece of unbleached cotton (butter muslin or tightly woven cheesecloth), or a basket-style paper coffee filter. Secure with a string, a rubber band, or a threaded metal canning band. This is to keep out fruit flies.

8. Place on your counter or in another spot that is 75° to 86°F/25° to 30°C. Stir with a wooden spoon now and then, if you remember. After 1 week, add the raw vinegar to the mixture. Continue to let it sit in the warm space, stirring if you want to. When you remove the cover, you may see a film developing on top. It is the beginning of the vinegar mother.

9. Check the vinegar in a month, when you should have nice acidity. However, it may take an additional month or two to fully develop. Test the pH: It should be 4.0 or below.

10. Bottle the finished vinegar, saving the mother for another batch or sharing with a friend. Use immediately or age to allow it to mellow and develop flavors.

QUINCE BUTTER

You can use the strained mash from this recipe to make quince butter. For every cup of mash, add sugar to taste, ¼ cup vinegar, ½ teaspoon ground cinnamon, and ¼ teaspoon each of ground cloves and allspice. Bring to a boil, reduce to a simmer, and cook until you reach the desired consistency, about 30 minutes. The butter will keep for a few months in the refrigerator.

Shallot Vinegar

SHALLOT VINAIGRETTE is one of the great salad dressings, so I thought a shallot vinegar might facilitate a "shalloty" dressing with or without shallots on hand. Sure enough, it is delicious and makes a great vinaigrette starter.

I do have to warn you, though: During the first week or two of fermentation, as the mixture is turning into alcohol, it has a very strong smell, like cooking shallots or gas. My husband, Christopher, was convinced our stove had a gas leak, but it was the shallots. I love the essence of the shallots and have not experimented further, but I assume you could substitute other types of onions for this recipe.

YIELD
about 1 quart

½ pound (226 g) shallots

Unchlorinated water

¼ cup (52 g) sugar, any kind

½ teaspoon (1 g) wine yeast hydrated in ¼ cup (59 mL) unchlorinated water, warmed to 104°F/40°C; or ½ cup (118 mL) room-temperature wild yeast starter (page 53)

½ cup (118 mL) raw, unfiltered, unpasteurized vinegar, or a vinegar mother

1. If you have a juicer, you can run the shallots through the juicer. Otherwise, chop the shallots, put them into a blender, and purée. Transfer the shallot juice or mash to a sanitized quart jar. Add enough water to reach the 3-cup mark.

2. Add the sugar and stir.

3. Stir in the hydrated yeast or wild yeast starter.

4. Stir the mixture well with a wooden spoon. Unlike with most ferments, you want to get oxygen in the mix. However, make sure the shallot mash stays submerged; otherwise it can become a host for undesirable opportunistic bacteria.

5. Cover the jar with a piece of unbleached cotton (butter muslin or tightly woven cheesecloth), or a basket-style paper coffee filter. Secure with a string, a rubber band, or a threaded metal canning band. This is to keep out fruit flies.

6. Place on your counter at room temperature.

7. Stir once a day for the first 5 or 6 days. You may see bubbles: That is good. After 5 or 6 days, if you have fermenting juice, proceed to step 8. If you have a mash, line a strainer with a piece of butter muslin or fine-mesh cheesecloth and strain the mixture into a new sanitized jar. Press on the mash and squeeze the cloth to

get every last tasty drop out. (Use this shallot mash to flavor butter or oil when sautéing. It's a great fried rice starter.)

8. Add the vinegar. Now keep the almost-vinegar a bit warmer, by placing it in a spot that is 75° to 86°F/25° to 30°C.

9. Check the vinegar in a month, when you should have nice acidity. However, it may take another month or two to fully develop, especially if your environment is cooler.

10. Bottle the finished vinegar. Use immediately, or age for a few months and use within the first year; this vinegar doesn't benefit from long aging.

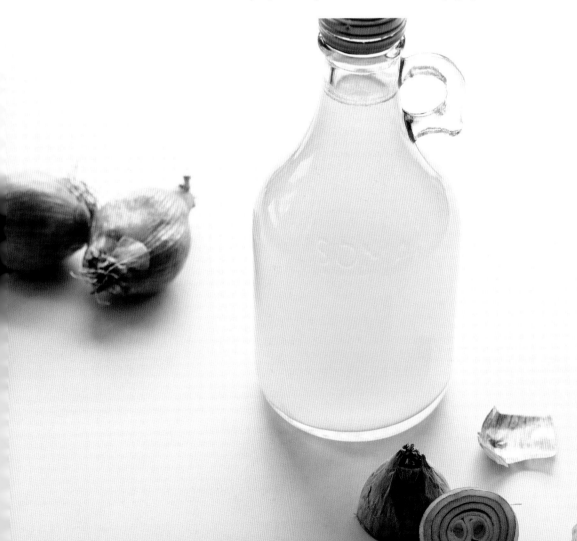

Tomato Vinegar

THIS VINEGAR REMINDS ME of liquid sun-dried tomatoes. It is pure summer garden in a jar. Sprinkle this on a dish and forget about needing out-of-season tomatoes; you will get so much more tomato flavor here. On a practical level, if you're a gardener, or if you have access to a lot of tomatoes during that beautiful time that is fresh tomato season, this is a quick, easy way to process some of that abundance. And it doesn't involve standing over a hot, steaming pot of roasting tomatoes or canning jars.

The recipe here ferments the tomatoes in an open jar. Use tomatoes that are very ripe; overripe is also fine. They should be unblemished, so cut off any bruises or bad parts. Alternatively, using a vacuum sealer to make tomato vinegar is even easier (see page 159).

(see page 159)

**YIELD
about 1½
quarts**

1¾–2 pounds (794–907 g) ripe tomatoes

1. Put the tomatoes in a sanitized half-gallon jar, leaving 2 inches of headspace below the neck, mashing the tomatoes well as you fill to press out air pockets.

2. Cover the jar with a piece of unbleached cotton (butter muslin or tightly woven cheesecloth), or a basket-style paper coffee filter. Secure with a string, a rubber band, or a threaded metal canning band. This is to keep out fruit flies.

3. Set your vessel in a warm (ideally, 75° to 86°F/25° to 30°C) and visible spot, so that you won't forget it. You will need to stir it often for the first few weeks to build flavor and work out air pockets that if left too long can develop mold. I suggest stirring every day, because then you can build it into your routine. (Drink your coffee, stir your mushy vinegar baby . . .)

4. The mixture will soften, then turn effervescent. After the initial fermentation calms down, let the batch rest. It should be ready in 2 to 3 months.

5. For a pulpy vinegar, strain the mixture with a wide-mesh strainer to remove just the seeds and skin. For a clearer vinegar, allow the pulp to settle out (refrigerating will help this along) and rack the clear vinegar off the top. (Use the pulp in sauces, soups, and cooking. Whatever you do, don't toss it—it is so tasty.)

6. Bottle the finished vinegar. Use immediately, or age to allow it to mellow and develop flavors. The next time you make this recipe, add ¼ cup (59 mL) of the finished vinegar in step 1, to give it a solid start.

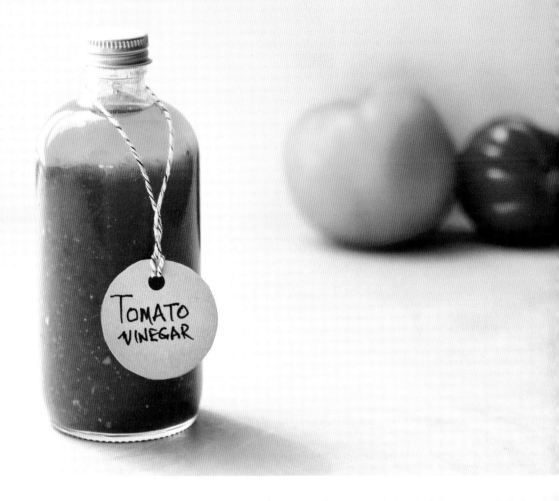

TRY THIS: VACUUM-SEALED VINEGAR

An alternative method for making tomato vinegar is to simply vacuum seal unblemished, clean, whole ripe tomatoes in a bag. Jot down the date on the bag, and set the bag aside. I have forgotten one of my bags for nearly two years (recommended!). When the tomatoes have liquefied, cut open the bag and pour the contents into a jar. This liquid is an amazing elixir and can be used immediately. Its sourness comes from the lactic acid bacteria, which can thrive in anaerobic environments. It is extremely tasty; you can simply strain out the skins and use it as is. Keep it refrigerated if you stop here.

At this point, you can add a little raw vinegar and oxygen to continue the fermentation on the last of the carbohydrates, which will make the product more stable. Strain out the skins, pour the liquid into a jar, add a tablespoon of raw vinegar, and cover the jar with a piece of tightly woven cloth secured with a rubber band. Let it ferment for another month, then enjoy. You may strain out the solids or rack off the clear vinegar, but I like to keep all the pulp and tomato goodness intact.

This method is also wonderful for persimmons and other soft, juicy fruits. For fruit with lower sugar values, add sugar to the bag (refer to the amounts listed on page 162) before you vacuum seal it.

Universal Country-Style Fruit Wine Vinegar

COUNTRY WINE IS A TERM often used for alcoholic beverages made from flowers (think dandelion wine), fruits, or vegetables, instead of grapes. Vinegar recipes that are not apple cider vinegars, wine vinegars, rice vinegars, or other traditional vinegars are often based on country wines. Some country wine recipes contain significantly less sugar than what I call for here. That's because this is a general recipe, and the amount of sugar listed will ensure enough alcohol and then acid development without your having to measure specific gravity or Brix. Any type of sugar will work; I generally use raw cane sugar, but regular white sugar works well. You can also use a variety of different aromatic herbs to build flavor; herb quantities vary depending on how potent the herb is, but I generally use 2 to 9 grams of each type.

YIELD
about 1 quart

1 pound (454 g) fruit and/or vegetables

Aromatic botanicals (optional)

Juice of 1 lemon

5 cups (1.2 L) water

1 pound (454 g) sugar, any kind

½ teaspoon (1 g) wine yeast hydrated in ¼ cup (59 mL) unchlorinated water, warmed to 104°F/40°C; or ½ cup (118 mL) room-temperature wild yeast starter (page 53)

1 cup (237 mL) raw, unfiltered, unpasteurized vinegar, or a vinegar mother

1. Clean the fruit and/or vegetables, and the botanicals, if using. Remove and discard the stems from fruit. For most types of flowers, add only the petals. Mash or grate the fruit or vegetables. Place the plant material, along with the lemon juice, in a sanitized half-gallon jar or other fermentation container.

2. Combine the water and sugar in a large pot and bring to a boil, stirring until the sugar is dissolved. Pour the boiling sugar water into the fruit or vegetable mix. Cover and let steep for about 48 hours, stirring a few times a day.

3. Remove the large pieces of plant material and strain the liquid through cheesecloth. Squeeze the cloth to extract as much of the flavorful juice as possible. Return to the same jar or a new, sanitized jar. Make sure this "tea" is at room temperature.

4. Add the hydrated yeast liquid or the wild yeast starter to the jar. Stir well with a wooden spoon.

5. Cover the jar with a piece of unbleached cotton (butter muslin or tightly woven cheesecloth), or a basket-style paper coffee filter. Secure with a string, a rubber band, or a threaded metal canning band. This is to keep out fruit flies.

6. Stir with a wooden spoon now and then, if you remember. You may see bubbles: That is good. The ferment will begin to slow down in about 2 weeks.

7. When the fermentation has slowed, add the vinegar and stir. Replace the cover and set the jar on your counter or in another spot that is 75° to 86°F/25° to 30°C. Again, stir if you think about it, to oxygenate. When you remove the cover, you may see a film developing on top. This is the beginning of the vinegar mother.

8. Check the vinegar in a month, when you should have nice acidity. However, it may take another month or two to fully develop, especially if your environment is cooler. The pH should be 4.0 or below.

9. Bottle the finished vinegar, saving the mother for another batch or sharing with a friend. Use immediately, or age to allow it to mellow and develop flavors.

RECIPES AS ROAD MAPS

As you may have noticed, many of the recipes in this book are both a recipe and an example of a process, as well as an invitation to try the method with your own ideas and ingredients. These include Universal Wine Vinegar (page 129), Universal Country-Style Fruit Wine Vinegar (page 160), Universal Wild Whole-Fruit Vinegar (page 162), Universal Scrap Vinegar (page 192), and Universal Amazake Scrap Vinegar (page 195). Think of them as recipe road maps for anything that comes your way, whether it's wildcrafted goodies or garden abundance. This adventure is yours, and you can choose your own path, whether you're working with chanterelles or ramps or huckleberries or cactus fruit.

Universal Wild Whole-Fruit Vinegar

THIS IS A WONDERFUL WAY to make vinegar when you have an abundance of soft fruit, like berries and stone fruits. Pome fruits do better with juicing. You can also use fruit that is too ripe to eat—a little fermentation is fine, but be sure to remove any dark bruises or mold. Like with the Japanese Persimmon Vinegar (page 150) or Brown Banana Vinegar (page 178), you are simply letting nature take its course. These vinegars are a pure expression of the life of fruit, and the flavors are fantastic. Be aware that some fruit does not contain enough inherent sugar to produce a high enough ABV. In the recipe below, you'll find sugar amounts that correspond with different types of fruit. Use any type of sugar; I generally use raw cane sugar, but regular white sugar also works well and is less expensive.

You can add aromatic botanicals or herbs to this mash. Taste it as the mixture ferments, and remove these extras whenever the flavor is to your liking.

YIELD
varies by
fruit used

2 quarts (around 1.9 kg) mashed blackberries, blueberries, fresh currants, elderberries, melons, raspberries, chokecherries, or gooseberries and 1 cup (200 g) sugar, any kind

or

2 quarts (around 1.9 kg) mashed kiwifruit, papaya, or mangoes and ½ cup (100 g) sugar

or

2 quarts (around 1.9 kg) mashed apricots, cherries, or peaches and ⅓ cup (67 g) sugar

or

2 quarts (around 1.9 kg) grapes or plums, with no added sugar

1. Layer the fruit in a sanitized half-gallon (or larger) jar, sprinkling in the appropriate amount of sugar as you go. Mash the fruit and sugar mixture well, pressing out air pockets.

2. Cover the jar with a piece of unbleached cotton (butter muslin or tightly woven cheesecloth), or a basket-style paper coffee filter. Secure with a string, a rubber band, or a threaded metal canning band. This is to keep out fruit flies.

3. Set your vessel in a warm (ideally 75° to 86°F/25° to 30°C), visible spot so that you won't forget it. You will need to stir it often for the first few weeks to build flavor and work out air pockets that if left too long can develop mold. I suggest stirring every day, because then you can build it into your routine. (Drink your coffee, stir your mushy vinegar baby . . .)

4. The mixture will soften, then turn effervescent. After the initial fermentation calms down, let the batch rest for about 3 months, until it's ready to strain.

5. Line a strainer with a piece of butter muslin or fine-mesh cheesecloth and strain the mixture into a new sanitized jar. Press on the fruit and squeeze the cloth to get every last tasty drop out.

6. Bottle the finished vinegar. Use immediately, or age to allow it to mellow and develop flavors. The next time, you can use some of this as a starter and it will help the new batch move a little bit faster.

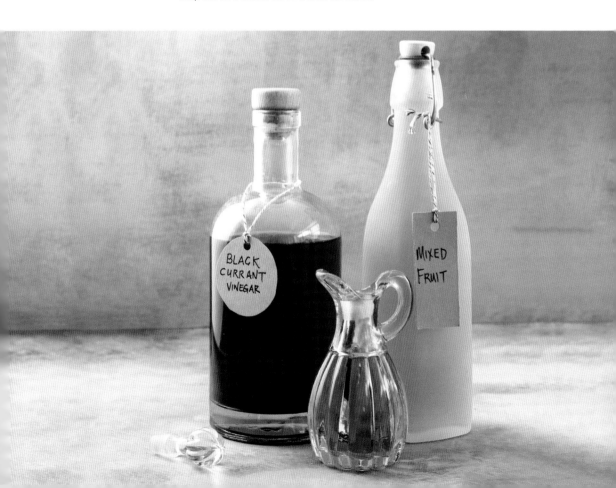

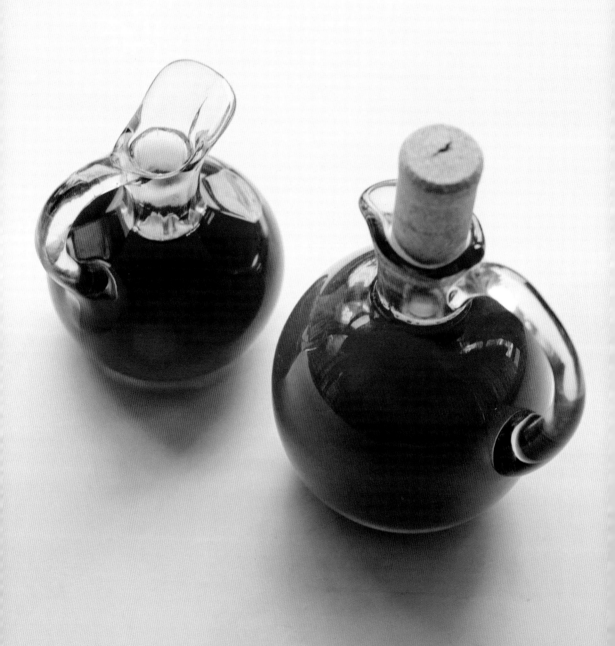

Purple Sweet Potato Vinegar

THIS PRETTY FUCHSIA VINEGAR, *benimosu*, is a traditional vinegar of Japan. That should come as no surprise, since sweet potatoes are used to produce alcohol there, the most common of which is shochu.

Only recently have purple sweet potatoes started showing up in markets across the United States, but these colored gems have been grown for a long time. Native to southern Central America and Colombia are ones with brown, red-orange, or white skin with orange or white flesh. The variety called Stokes Purple cooks up a little drier and denser than the white- or orange-fleshed ones commonly found at the market, which works well for growing koji (though the other varieties will work also). The other bonus is the purple pigment doesn't cook out or ferment away as happens with so many other purple vegetables. This means it stays beautiful, and the anthocyanins (the superantioxidant found in purple fruits and vegetables) and related phenolic compounds that may have beneficial health effects don't go away. In fact, making vinegar boosts all these good compounds, giving this ferment a higher antioxidative activity than other vinegars, including black vinegar (see page 85).[9]

YIELD
about 3 quarts

4 cups (700 g) sweet potato koji (instructions for growing koji on page 277) made from about 1½ pounds or 2 medium, fresh sweet potatoes

2.2 pounds (1 kg) chopped purple sweet potatoes (7–8 cups)

7 cups (1.7 L) unchlorinated water, warmed to 135°F/57°C

½ teaspoon (1 g) sake or wine yeast, hydrated in ¼ cup (59 mL) unchlorinated water that has been warmed to 104°F/40°C

½ cup (118 mL) raw, unfiltered, unpasteurized vinegar, or a vinegar mother

1. Begin the koji (see page 277) 24 to 30 hours before you want to start the vinegar.

2. Once the koji is ready, you will be making a sweet potato amazake. Put the chopped purple sweet potatoes in a large pot and top with the warm water. Simmer over medium heat until soft. Remove from the heat and let cool to 135°F/57°C.

3. Add the koji potatoes to the cooled potato and water mixture. Using a handheld blender, or processing the mixture in a blender in batches, purée the mixture until as smooth as possible.

recipe continues on next page

4. Transfer the mixture to a sanitized vessel and set in an incubation chamber or sous vide water bath set at a temperature between 135° and 138°F/57° and 59°C. Incubate the mixture for 6 to 10 hours or until it has a floral aroma and a mild, sweet taste. (The cooler the incubation, the longer it will take.) Stir the mixture after the first hour and again once or twice during incubation. If you want it sweeter and a little more liquidy, let it ferment a little longer. It will continue to sweeten, but only up to a point. When it hits its limit, the flavor will start to turn slightly sour and have some bitter or alcoholic notes.

5. When it is ready, cool it to around 100°F/38°C, then add the hydrated yeast to the now amazake. Stir it in. Let ferment for 48 hours or more, keeping it at room temperature.

6. After 48 hours of fermentation, there should be little yeast activity (heavy bubbling) remaining. Transfer the amazake to a clean crock or other open fermentation vessel. Stir in the vinegar.

7. Cover the crock with muslin or any cloth that will allow air circulation. Secure the cloth around the rim with a string or rubber band. Ferment on your counter or in another warm spot, ideally at 75° to 86°F/25° to 30°C. Stir daily for the first 2 weeks. Then let the fermentation continue for 6 weeks to 3 months, stirring occasionally. Check regularly; if surface yeast begins to form, continue to stir regularly. If surface yeast becomes a problem, you can spritz with 80 proof alcohol. Read more about this in the troubleshooting section on page 274. The vinegar is finished when it tastes brightly acidic; pH should be 4.0 or below.

8. If you plan to strain it, put in the refrigerator to settle the solids; this is called cold crashing. You can rack off the clear liquid first if you'd like. Strain the vinegar through a fine-mesh strainer or food mill to remove the thicker lees, leave the vinegar cloudy, or allow the lees to settle and rack off the clear purple vinegar: It's your choice. Save the lees (see Using Those Lees, opposite).

9. Bottle the finished vinegar. Use immediately, or age to continue to build and smooth flavors.

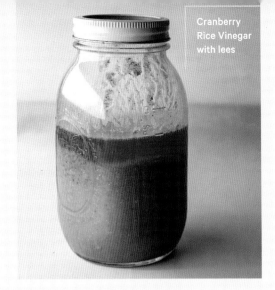
Cranberry
Rice Vinegar
with lees

USING THOSE LEES

The lees at the bottom of a starch-based vinegar are often quite delicious. Don't toss them out! Here are four ways to enjoy them—sweet or savory.

Sauce or butter. The puréed lees can be cooked gently in an open pot and reduced to an applesauce or apple butter consistency. Taste as you are cooking. It may be delicious as is, or you may want to add your favorite spices and sweetener for sweet-and-sour chutney flavors. Use this as a spread or as a condiment to dip tasty things in.

Snack leather. Take this rich cooked-down purée and spread it on dehydrator trays lined with parchment paper or fruit leather sheets. Dehydrate at 135°F/57°C for 8 to 10 hours.

Jam. With lees that have been made with fruit, you can make jam. The acidity of the lees brings out a lot of flavor; you'll simply add your sweetener to achieve the flavor you love. Here's my method: Place the puréed lees in an open-topped pot to simmer with the sugar and pectin. Plan to use ½ cup (100 grams) to 1 cup (200 grams) sweetener (to desired sweetness) and 1 teaspoon Pomona's pectin (see Note, below right) for every cup (200 grams) of purée. Measure the sugar or other sweetener into a bowl. If using a syrup, it should be at room temperature. Thoroughly mix the pectin powder in and set the mixture aside. Bring the fruit lees to a full boil. Add the pectin-sweetener mixture, and stir vigorously for 1 to 2 minutes to dissolve the pectin as the "jam" comes back to a boil. Once at a full boil, remove it from the heat. Transfer to clean jars and freeze or refrigerate.

In the refrigerator, the jams last 3 weeks. Use on toast, in thumbprint cookies, as a glaze . . .

Pickles. These lees are acidic and can be used much in the same way sake lees are used in traditional Japanese *kasuzuke* fermented pickles.

1. Place the thickly sliced vegetables in a container, such as a small plastic tub or casserole dish, that you will be able to apply a lot of weight to. Sprinkle the vegetables liberally with salt.

2. Cover the dish with plastic wrap or a clean cotton cloth. On top of this, place something heavy, such as a pot of water, a crock, or a tub of flour. Allow the vegetables to weep for 2 days. At that point, they should be limp.

3. Use the vinegar lees "straight" or combine with some salt, sugar, and spices to taste.

4. Cover the bottom of your fermentation vessel with the lees mixture, place the vegetables on top, and cover with another layer of the lees, making sure the vegetables are all tucked in and submerged. If your vessel is narrow, you may need to create several layers of lees and vegetables. Cover the container with plastic wrap or a clean cotton cloth, then weight it down.

5. Let the vegetables ferment for a few hours to a few days. Make sure that the vegetables stay submerged. They are done when you like them.

6. To serve, either lightly wipe off the lees to retain some of the flavor, or rinse the vegetables off.

NOTE: For years I've used Pomona's Universal Pectin, as it yields a firmer set. This is especially great for relatively low-sugar jams.

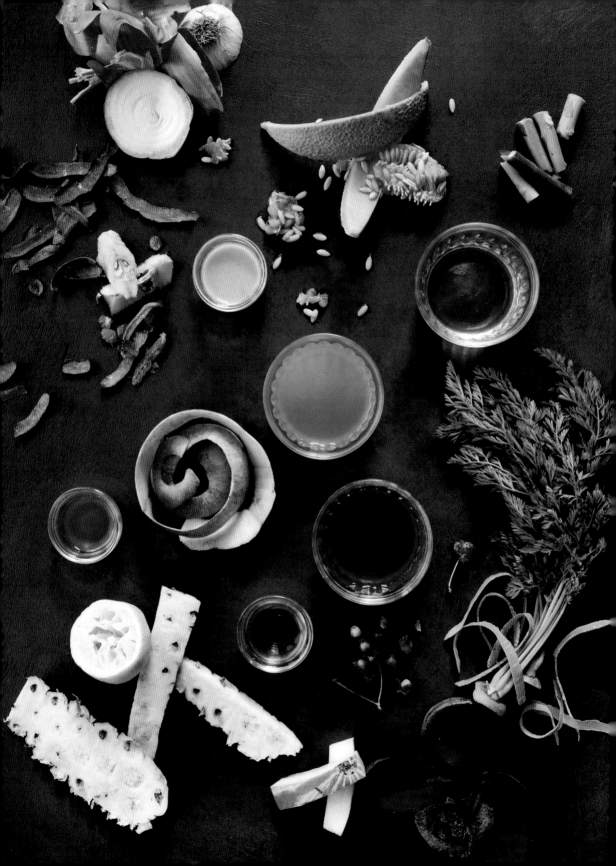

CHAPTER 7

VINEGARS FROM SCRAPS AND LEAVINGS

 ASTE NOT, WANT NOT is a proverb that drove the actions of the average American from this country's founding—that is, until the post–World War II years, when we tossed out this way of life as old-fashioned and ushered in decades of consumerism, TV dinners, and wasted food. The rest of the world followed our lead.

Fortunately, in recent years, there has been a growing effort to end food waste, not only in fields, factories, and restaurants, but also in our own kitchens. I am most excited about the potential vinegar has to glean enchanting flavored acid from food scraps that were formerly headed to the waste stream. Not only will you extract delicious nutrition from peelings and other leavings, but you will never need to buy expensive gourmet or raw vinegars.

STARTING WITH APPLE CORES

At the beginning of my family's homestead-ing adventure, I preserved anything that wasn't nailed down. It's no wonder that when I read *Farmer Boy* again as an adult and came across a line about apple core vinegar, I was intrigued. Armed with the Foxfire books and Carla Emery's *The Encyclopedia of Country Living*, but not the internet, I got closer to figuring out how to make this happen. The next time we had mounds of raw peelings and cores from making dried apple rings, I made my first vinegar—a fruit scrap vinegar. It was okay, but not great. Christopher and I began to make hard cider, but I had yet to understand fully the role of microbes and the importance of sugar in this transformation.

Honestly, it would be a few years before I would intentionally try to make vinegar. We were under the impression, as most fledgling home wine or cider makers are, that vinegar is something to be avoided. That it is a mistake or fault to judge yourself against. It was in moving beyond this thinking that I began my vinegar making. At that time, there was only one vinegar-specific book I could find (*Vinegar* by Lawrence J. Diggs) and still limited internet information.

It wasn't until this moment of intention that it clicked—I needed a decent alcohol for a good vinegar. I'd never made that connection with those first scrap vinegars. The cores and peels themselves didn't have enough sugar and nutri-ents to feed the yeast and bacteria sufficiently. Basically, the apple bathwater—or infusion, if you will, of scraps—needs a sugar boost for the yeast to create enough ethanol for a rich, sour vinegar.

Depending on your apple varieties, or other fruit, vegetable, or grain leavings, these scrap vinegars may or may not have enough sugar. If you are experimenting with your own fruit scrap vinegars, you have two choices: You can add sugar to be safe, or you can take a specific gravity measurement and add sugar only as needed. In most of the following recipes, instead of adding yeast (some old-school recipes add bread yeast to begin the process), you'll let the wild yeasts that are already on the fruit skins go to work.

VINEGAR AS AN EXAMPLE OF WHOLE UTILIZATION

Our society's thinking around reducing waste has changed over the last thirty years. In the late 1980s and 1990s, the buzzwords were REDUCE, REUSE, RECYCLE—themes that I worked into my curriculums as I was getting my degree in elementary education. In the early 2000s, the idea of "cradle to cradle" emerged: a closed-loop manufacturing process in which resources are recycled or reused rather than being dis-carded. At that time my husband, Christopher, landed what he thought would be his dream job, helping to create a cradle-to-cradle system at a small division within Hewlett-Packard. Zero waste came next: a principled way of living and manufacturing that focuses on design to reduce waste and recycle materials. The idea was to move materials through a pipeline with no waste on the back end.

The current thinking is that "whole utilization" may be the most realistic option; it's the idea that food will be used from nose to tail (or tip to root, if you prefer), but in the end, if there is some waste it makes it into a compost heap. Jori Jayne Emde, whom you will meet on page 182, doesn't believe zero waste is even possible. She's built her business around whole utilization. For vinegar, this practice works well, because many of these scrap vinegars pull the final nutrients, flavors, and life out of the peelings and bits—but ultimately there may be a stringy flavorless mash that ends up being composted.

Capturing the flavor of fruit scraps is one more way to use them before sending them to the compost pile. This vinegar used melon peels in amazake to create a delicious vinegar.

Apple Pomace Vinegar

THIS IS A simultaneous fermentation. The yeasts will still turn the sugar into ethanol, while the acetobacters, dropped in with the addition of raw vinegar, will be waiting in the wings to get started. As for the sugar, it is yeast food, so it doesn't matter what you use—white sugar or molasses or honey. The yeasts don't care. That said, while white sugar will keep the flavor neutral, like you would expect with an apple cider vinegar, molasses or honey will impart their own flavors to your final vinegar.

YIELD
1½ quarts

1 pound (450 g) apple mash from pressing

¾ cup (155 g) sugar, any kind

2 quarts (1.9 L) unchlorinated water, just off the boil

½ cup (118 mL) raw, unfiltered, unpasteurized vinegar, or a vinegar mother

1. Combine the fruit and sugar into a sanitized half-gallon jar. Add 1 quart of the just-boiled water. Use the remaining hot water to fill the jar to the neck.

2. When the water cools to room temperature, add the raw vinegar. Stir well with a wooden spoon. Unlike with most ferments, you want to get some oxygen into the mix. However, make sure the fruit scraps themselves stay submerged; otherwise they can become a host for undesirable opportunistic bacteria.

3. Cover the jar with a piece of unbleached cotton (butter muslin or tightly woven cheesecloth), or a basket-style paper coffee filter. Secure with a string, a rubber band, or a threaded metal canning band. This is to keep out fruit flies.

4. Place on your counter or in another spot that is 75° to 86°F/25° to 30°C.

5. Stir with a wooden spoon once a day for the first 5 or 6 days. After that, stir now and then, if you remember. You may see bubbles: That is good.

6. The ferment will begin to slow down in about 2 weeks, at which point it's time to take out the scraps. When you remove the cover, you may see a film developing on top. It is the beginning of the vinegar mother. Remove and set it aside while you're straining out the fruit solids.

7. Line a strainer with a piece of butter muslin or fine-mesh cheesecloth and strain the mixture into a new sanitized jar. Press on the fruit and squeeze the cloth to get every last tasty drop out. Add the mother (if you have one) back into the jar and cover again.

8. Check the vinegar in a month, when you should have nice acidity. However, it may take an additional month or two to fully develop. Test the pH: It should be 4.0 or below.

9. Bottle the finished vinegar, saving the mother for another batch or sharing with a friend. Use immediately, or age to allow it to mellow and develop flavors.

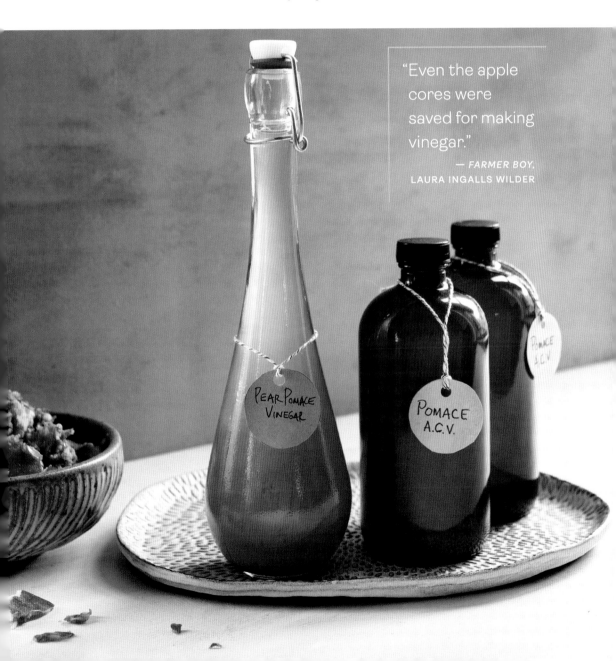

"Even the apple cores were saved for making vinegar."

— *FARMER BOY,*
LAURA INGALLS WILDER

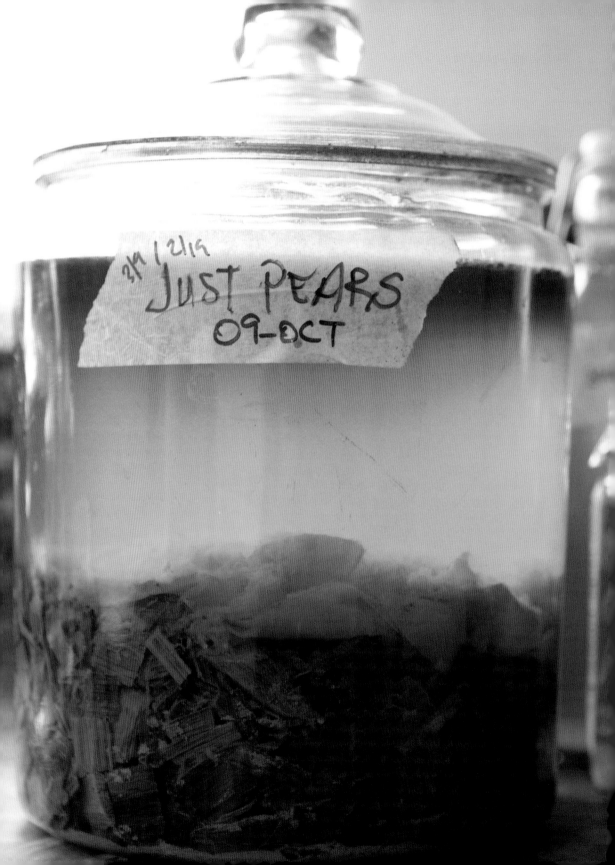

Variation:
Pear Pomace Vinegar

AT THE EDGE of our garden is an old Seckel pear tree that was likely planted in the 1940s or earlier. It's still vigorous and well formed, producing hundreds of the sweet, small, rusty-red-blushed fruit this variety is known for. Over the years, we've made dried pears, steamed pear juice, pear butter, and pear crisps with these small fruits. They have also been added to the annual cider-pressing bins. Only more recently did we begin to make a perry that is mostly these Seckels with a bit of a supersharp tannic pear. A few years ago, I couldn't bear to toss the pomace. Unlike pressed apples that come out very dry, the squeezed pears seemed to have a lot of goodness still left in them. Turns out they did. It was the best pear vinegar we'd ever tasted— well, it might have also been the first. We now make this every year and use it all year long in soda water.

The apple pomace vinegar recipe on page 172 also works with any type of pear. Follow the instructions for that recipe, but omit the sugar. That's right—the beauty of this vinegar is that it's simply pomace and water. We've made it with sugar to test the process, and it comes out much more delicious without it.

Asparagus Vinegar

FRESH ASPARAGUS SEASON is one of my favorites. I look forward to those sweet shoots, and I miss them when they're gone. I'm always trying to figure out how to use the woody ends. This vinegar is sweet and tastes just like fresh asparagus drenched in lemon juice. Often a pile of ends will yield enough juice. If it doesn't, go ahead and use some stalks as well. And I won't tell if you run to the market and buy the whole stalks to make this from the get-go.

YIELD
about 1 quart

2 pounds (907 g) woody asparagus ends

Room-temperature unchlorinated water to make 5 cups (1.2 L) asparagus juice

¾ cup (175 g) sugar, any kind

½ teaspoon (1 g) wine yeast hydrated in ¼ cup (59 mL) unchlorinated water, warmed to 104°F/40°C; or ½ cup (118 mL) room-temperature wild yeast starter (page 53)

½ cup (118 mL) raw, unfiltered, unpasteurized vinegar, or a vinegar mother

1. Run the asparagus through a juicer or chop it and blend it in a blender. Put the asparagus mash in a straining bag or cheesecloth and squeeze out all of the juice. Transfer the juice to a sanitized half-gallon jar. Add room temperature unchlorinated water until you have 5 cups of liquid.

2. Add the sugar and stir.

3. Add the hydrated yeast liquid or the wild yeast starter to the jar.

4. Add the vinegar. Stir well with a wooden spoon. Unlike with most ferments, you want to get oxygen into the mix.

5. Cover the jar with a piece of unbleached cotton (butter muslin or tightly woven cheesecloth), or a basket-style paper coffee filter. Secure with a string, a rubber band, or a threaded metal canning band. This is to keep out fruit flies.

6. Place on your counter or in another spot that is 75° to 86°F/25° to 30°C.

7. Stir once a day for the first 5 or 6 days. You may stir it occasionally after that, but because this vinegar has always created a good mother, I generally don't. Check the vinegar in a month, when you should have nice acidity. However, it may take another month or two to fully develop, especially if your environment is cooler.

8. Bottle the finished vinegar, saving the mother for another batch or sharing with a friend. Use immediately, or age to allow it to mellow and develop flavors.

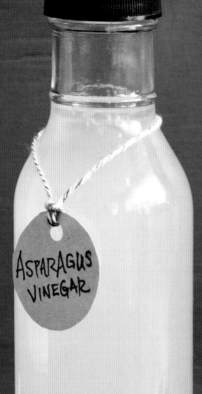
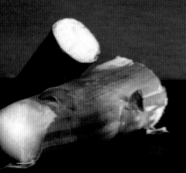

Brown Banana Vinegar

I ADMIT TO NOT BEING a huge banana eater as an adult—despite my lingering deep enjoyment of fried bananas. They are just not a go-to for me. Now that the kids are grown, Christopher and I have a running (quirky) routine: He buys bananas, and I roll my eyes. We both know I won't eat them, and he loves them but rarely finishes the cluster he brings home before they get browner and browner, full of squishy sugar. Then I step in and freeze them—for vinegar.

In this recipe, you will use dark brown, even black, bananas. You can either allow a number of bananas to blacken (leave them in a warm spot for a few days) or save just the one or two that get overripe, peeled and frozen until you have enough. I have made this vinegar with unpeeled (organic) mashed black bananas as well. The results were unpredictable. When it worked, the flavor had a bit of a bitter but tasty dimension. It also got sour a little sooner, likely due to all the extra yeast and microbes on the peel. In repeated trials, the final product was tastier and more consistent when the bananas were peeled.

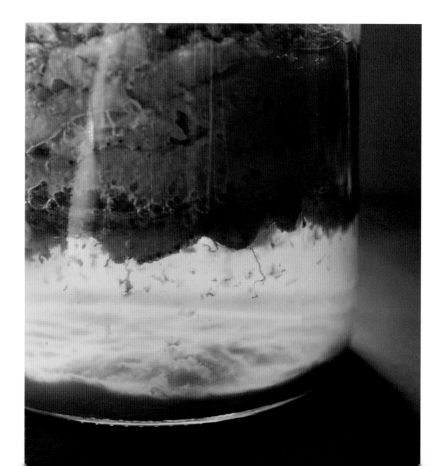

YIELD
½ to 1 pint

10–12 overripe bananas

2–3 tablespoons (29–44 mL) raw, unfiltered, unpasteurized vinegar

1. Peel the bananas and purée the pulp in a blender or a food processor. Alternatively, use a potato masher until you have a smooth mashed paste. Chop up the peels and toss them in your compost heap.

2. Transfer the mash to a sanitized quart jar. Cover the jar with a piece of unbleached cotton (butter muslin or tightly woven cheesecloth), or a basket-style paper coffee filter. Secure with a string, a rubber band, or a threaded metal canning band. This is to keep out fruit flies.

3. You will see the banana mash begin to liquefy. The layer of future vinegar will be on the bottom with the pulp on top. For the first few days, stir daily to mix the top back in. This will keep surface fungi from forming.

4. After 4 or 5 days, when you see this liquid/pulp separation, allow the two layers to form and pour a small amount of raw vinegar on top. The pulp layer should be thick enough to allow this addition to stay on top. Note that this vinegar is not added to inoculate the mixture but to help the surface form a skin that will withstand surface growth as you let the bananas age and sour. Alternatively, you can simply keep stirring daily throughout the fermentation period. Allow to separate before bottling. The vinegar is ready when the flavor is punchy and acidic. The pH should be 4.0 or below.

5. Since the pulp separates, it is easy to pour off the clear vinegar. Bottle the finished vinegar. Transfer the fermented, acidic pulp to an airtight container and store it in the fridge until you're ready to make banana bread; it will last at least a few weeks.

ORIGINS OF BANANA VINEGAR

I first encountered banana vinegar in Costa Rica, and it rocked my world. It was pure banana but deliciously sour. Unfortunately, at the time it didn't occur to me to ask how it was made, but I did bring some home. When I ran out of that small bottle, I began using the overripe bananas according to my method for scrap vinegar. The vinegar was super tasty but not quite the rich, amber liquid I'd brought home. Then through social media, someone shared that they lived on an organic farm in Costa Rica where they made vinegar in the traditional farm style by hanging the entire banana bunch in a dark garage and covering it with a porous gunny sack. The whole thing ferments—bananas, skin and all. The resulting liquid that collects in a bag at the bottom is the vinegar. Since that initial aha moment, I have learned that in areas that grow bananas and plantains, these vinegars were historically made from the fruit that was getting overripe (brown) to preserve, and thus use, them. Depending on the region, methods varied from the hanging technique above to mashing the flesh to ferment it.

Fermented Banana Pulp Bread

WHEN YOUR BANANA VINEGAR is finished, you'll end up with extra pulp that is fermenty and delicious, and can still be used for making banana bread. The fermented banana mash is a deep, dark mush pulp—sludge, really. Alas, "banana sludge bread" just doesn't sound appealing, but don't let that deter you from making this recipe. The acidic fermented pulp is delicious and offers wonderful moisture and acidity that comes through in the bread.

YIELD
1 loaf

1 cup (120 g) all-purpose flour, plus more for the pan

1 teaspoon (5 g) baking powder

¼ teaspoon (1.2 g) baking soda

¼ teaspoon (1 g) salt

¼ teaspoon (1 g) grated nutmeg

1 egg

⅔ cup (120 g) coconut sugar

4 tablespoons (56 g) melted butter

¼ cup (59 mL) whole milk

⅔ cup (158 g) fermented banana pulp, from vinegar making

1. Preheat the oven to 350°F/180°C. Grease and flour an 8- by 4-inch loaf pan.

2. Sift or stir together the flour, baking powder, baking soda, salt, and nutmeg in a medium bowl.

3. In a large bowl, whisk the egg until it has a consistent golden color, then stir in the sugar, butter, and milk.

4. Pour the banana pulp into the egg mixture and stir with a silicone spatula to combine.

5. Sift about half of the flour mixture into the banana-egg mixture, gently folding to combine. You want to barely incorporate the flour so that the loaf will stay moist when baked. Add the remaining flour mixture and repeat the folding until just combined.

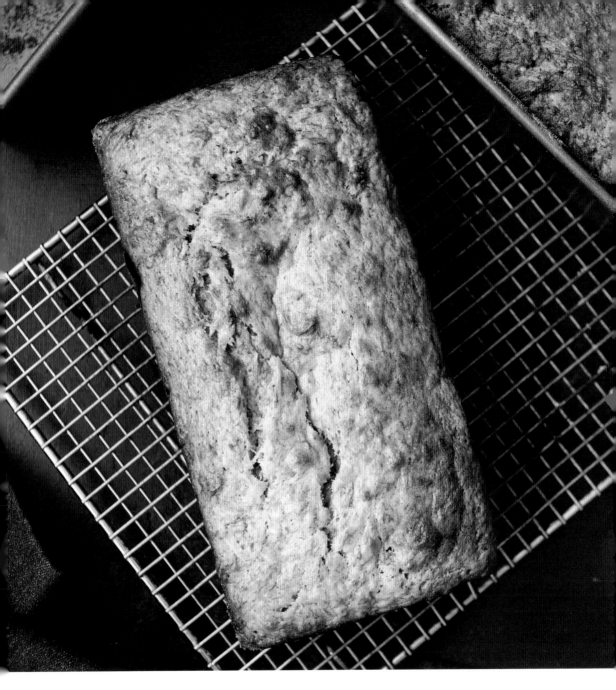

6. Pour the batter into the prepared pan. Bake for about 40 minutes, or until a toothpick inserted in the center comes out clean.

7. Set the pan on a wire rack to cool for a few minutes, then invert the pan to remove the loaf. Let that cool before eating—although when the bread is still warm, it melts a pat of butter to perfection.

LADY JAYNE'S ALCHEMY

Jori Jayne Emde describes herself as a flavor maven. From creating and maintaining the fermentation larder at Fish & Game—the James Beard Award–winning restaurant she founded in Hudson, New York, with her husband, Zakary Pelaccio—to bringing to life unique ferments for her company, Lady Jayne's Alchemy, Jori's passion for vinegar making developed out of her quest for deep, funky, fermented flavors.

Her passion is also driven by a desire to reduce food waste and a need to address health issues. She blames a high-sugar diet for her health issues, which started when she was a young adult, and credits vinegar (sugar's ultimate transformation) for healing her. Her early forays into fermentation were focused on making drinking vinegars for herself.

"For me [vinegar making] has always been more of a health quest," she says.

Today, she interacts with vinegar from head to toe: in her hair rinse; in the neti pot; via drinking vinegars for stomach ulcers, kidney stones, and female health; and in the household for cleaning and laundry.

Making vinegar also makes use of food waste from the restaurant. If there's a possibility of flavor left in something, Jori will use it—whether it's cherry pits, carrot peels, stale bread, or not-quite-empty bottles of wine. In fact, many of her vinegars are made by adding the kitchen-scrap ingredients to the leftover wine. All of her work is what she calls native fermentation, meaning no added yeasts and no infusions.

She also draws inspiration from an unusual place: old recipes written in medieval English. Reading these recipes doesn't translate into direct use in the kitchen. Instead, they lie dormant and are part of the well that feeds her intuition. (For example, an old random recipe that described making vinegar from a stale lump of bread and two apples inspired her to try making vinegar from cherry pits.)

Jori loves acid and the way it plays with food. She describes this work of creating flavor and acid as the "salt and pepper" of the operation. Here are a few pieces of advice, based on her years of fermenting experience.

UNDERSTAND YOUR INGREDIENTS— EVEN IF THEY'RE SCRAPS. If you make vinegar from the peelings of garden-grown carrots, it will be different from a vinegar made from commodity carrots. The fresh carrots from your garden are rich with nutrients, flavors, and fresh fermentable sugars; carrots from the grocery store will have fewer nutrients and less flavor, and long storage often leaves them starchy and dry in comparison, with fewer fermentable sugars (see page 138). That's not to say you shouldn't use commodity ingredients; just understand that using the best ingredients possible will result in a better end product.

SAVE YOUR WINE DREGS. Start a collection jar in your fridge, where you pour any old wine that's been open for too long or the sediment-laden dregs at the bottom of the bottle. You can separate the jars based on wine colors or simply have a general collection jar where any and all wine is collected and then used. When you've collected enough, start your vinegar fermentation; for example, Jori uses these to start her scrap vinegar. Alternatively, you could set up a continuous-brew pot for a rotating house vinegar (see page 90).

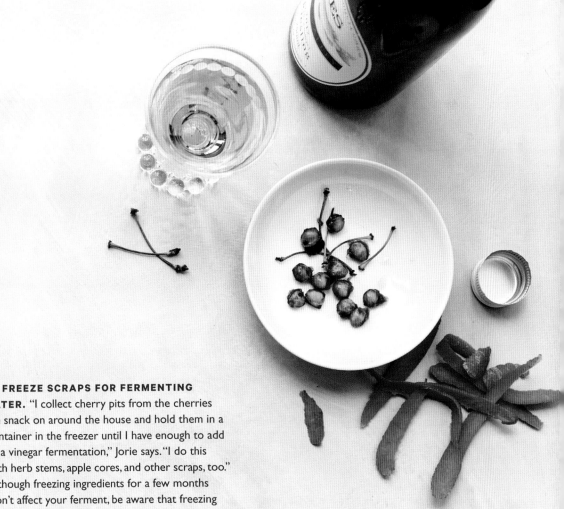

**FREEZE SCRAPS FOR FERMENTING
LATER.** "I collect cherry pits from the cherries
we snack on around the house and hold them in a
container in the freezer until I have enough to add
to a vinegar fermentation," Jorie says. "I do this
with herb stems, apple cores, and other scraps, too."
Although freezing ingredients for a few months
won't affect your ferment, be aware that freezing
them for a year or longer will kill the native yeasts,
making them not useful as the base from which to
make your starting alcohol. This isn't an issue if you
are adding the scraps to ready-made alcohol, since
you're not chasing the yeast to make it.

**TAP INTO YOUR INTUITION FOR PAIR-
ING FOODS.** Do you love apples and cinnamon?
Then why not pair apple peelings and cores with
cinnamon sticks in your vinegar ferment? Do you
love carrots and dill together? Then collect dill
stems and/or seeds to ferment with carrot peelings
and nubs. "The more you connect with what you
already know," Jori says, "the more confidence you'll
have. And with confidence comes the courage to
stretch beyond what you're comfortable with,
to reach for something new and adventurous."

DON'T TOSS IT! If you make a vinegar ferment
and you don't like the way it tastes, don't throw it
out. Just add a few drops of essential oil to the solution and use it as a natural, all-purpose cleaner. Or
add ¼ cup of vinegar to your load of laundry to act
as a natural fabric softener.

NEVER BE AFRAID TO SCREW UP. Mistakes
are inevitable (we're only human, after all), but making mistakes is a great way to refine skills. To track
your progress and analyze your inevitable failures,
keep a detailed log or journal regarding each project you start. Detailed notes are also helpful, Jori
says, "when you create something brilliant and want
to replicate it easily."

Corncob and Husk Vinegar

I TRIED AT LEAST a half-dozen ways to make a sweet corn vinegar, with results varying from "meh" to "ick" to "this isn't safe." (Don't worry, you will know if that ever happens to you—when the "wrong" microbes take over, it is 100 percent "yuck!" The result just smells rotten.) With each of those test batches, I was left with a pile of husks and cobs. And since there's still a lot of flavor in the husks and plenty of sugar left in the cob (the inside marrow of a raw cob is surprisingly sweet), I made vinegar. This recipe produces vinegar with a light corn flavor, but it's very harsh when first finished; age it for at least six months. In testing, I found that the starting "broth" always had some measurable sugar but needed more to bring the alcohol level into the right range. You might also notice the wild yeast starter isn't given as an option; for some reason this recipe always turned out much better with wine yeast.

For this recipe, I use 12 cobs, simply because our local corn stand (and maybe yours) still sells corn by the dozen. But feel free to adjust as needed. This recipe has worked again and again. My takeaway: Enjoy the kernels fresh and sweet, and make vinegar with the scraps.

YIELD
2 to 3 quarts

12 corncobs and their husks

3 quarts (2.8 L) room-temperature, unchlorinated water

2¼ cups (450 g) sugar, any kind

½ teaspoon (1 g) wine yeast hydrated in ¼ cup (59 mL) unchlorinated water, warmed to 104°F/40°C

2 cups (473 mL) raw vinegar with mother, if available, or vinegar from previous batch

1. Husk the corn, saving all the husks (the silk is fine, too) but removing any bits that are mildewed. Place the husks in a stockpot with the cool water and bring to a simmer.

2. Cut the corn kernels off the raw or cooked cobs. (Use the kernels in another recipe.) Cut the cobs into 2- to 3-inch chunks and add to the simmering husks. Simmer over low heat until the corn liquor is light gold in color and tastes like corn, 3 to 4 hours.

3. Remove the pot from the heat. When the mixture has cooled, line a strainer with a piece of butter muslin or fine-mesh cheesecloth and strain the mixture into a sanitized gallon jar. Be sure to wring out the husks, as they will hold on to a lot of your tasty liquor.

4. Ideally, at this point the jar will have at least 3 inches of headspace. Stir in the sugar, then add the hydrated yeast liquid. Stir well.

5. Cover the jar with a piece of unbleached cotton (butter muslin or tightly woven cheesecloth), or a basket-style paper coffee filter. Secure with a string, a rubber band, or a threaded metal canning band. This is to keep out fruit flies. Place on your counter or in another spot that is 75° to 86°F/25° to 30°C.

6. The next day, stir in the vinegar. Replace the cover and return the jar to its cozy spot.

7. In about 6 weeks, this vinegar will be quite acidic and harsh and it will likely have a mother. If the mother is thin, you can let the vinegar continue to age and mellow, or you can bottle the vinegar as is. When the mother becomes more vigorous, you will want to get the vinegar off the mother and out of the oxygenation process by bottling the liquid and saving the mother for another batch or sharing with a friend.

NOTE: Another good use for corncobs, either instead of making this vinegar or as a way to reuse the cobs after making vinegar from them, is as packing material in the kitchen-counter Boerhaave method of vinegar brewing (page 94).

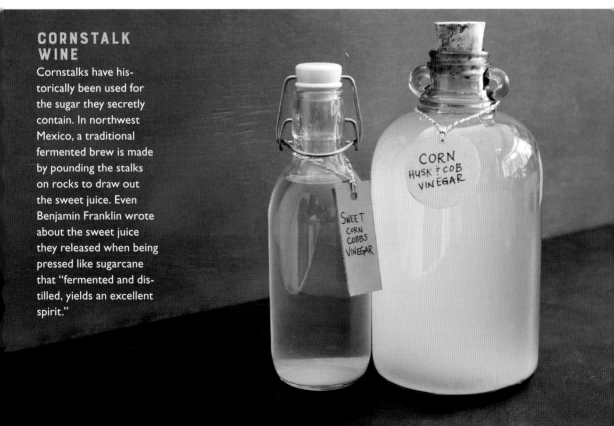

CORNSTALK WINE

Cornstalks have historically been used for the sugar they secretly contain. In northwest Mexico, a traditional fermented brew is made by pounding the stalks on rocks to draw out the sweet juice. Even Benjamin Franklin wrote about the sweet juice they released when being pressed like sugarcane that "fermented and distilled, yields an excellent spirit."

Grapefruit and Friends Scrap Vinegar

I PREPARE THIS RECIPE anytime I have citrus scraps, but the hands-down favorite versions in our household are the vinegars that are heavy on grapefruit skins. This recipe "cheats" a little by using one whole grapefruit. Feel free to use just the peels and bits, but I couldn't help myself—adding the extra was worth the grapefruit-forward flavor. I sprinkle this vinegar on salads, but its special spot is when I want a little acid added to a breakfast dish.

Don't fret if you can't eat the required amount of citrus in one sitting: You can collect scraps in the refrigerator until you have enough. Citrus holds up well in the fridge. I like to use at least a pound of these peels, but there is a lot of leeway in the method.

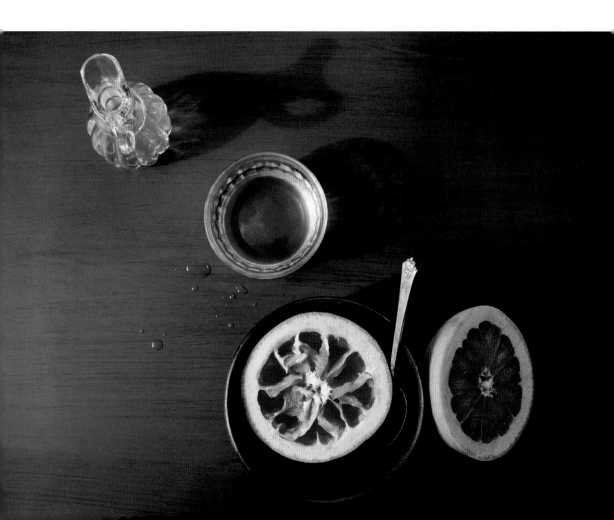

YIELD
about 2 quarts

1 pound (450 g) grapefruit rinds (or squeezed limes, or lemons, or a combination of the two), with pith and any pulp and juice left after eating or squeezing the juice

1 grapefruit, cut in half, with juice

¾ cup (155 g) sugar, any kind

1½ quarts (1.4 L) unchlorinated water, just off the boil

½ teaspoon (1 g) wine yeast hydrated in ¼ cup (59 mL) unchlorinated water that has been warmed to 104°F/40°C; or ½ cup (118 mL) room-temperature wild yeast starter (page 53)

¾ cup (177 mL) raw, unfiltered, unpasteurized vinegar, or a vinegar mother

1. Put the grapefruit rinds, plus the juice and rind of the whole fruit, with the sugar in a sanitized half-gallon jar. Stir in 1 quart of the just-boiled water. Use the rest of the water to fill the jar to the neck.

2. When the fruit mixture has cooled to room temperature, stir in the hydrated yeast liquid or the wild yeast. Stir well with a wooden spoon. You want to get some oxygen in the mix and make sure the fruit scraps themselves stay submerged; otherwise they can become a host for undesirable opportunistic bacteria.

3. Cover the jar with a piece of unbleached cotton (butter muslin or tightly woven cheesecloth), or a basket-style paper coffee filter. Secure with a string, a rubber band, or a threaded metal canning band. This is to keep out fruit flies.

4. Place on your counter or in another spot that is 75° to 86°F/25° to 30°C.

5. Stir once a day for the first 5 or 6 days. You may see bubbles: That is good. On day 5 or 6, stir in the vinegar. After that, stir with a wooden spoon now and then, especially if you see the scraps poking out of the liquid.

6. The ferment will begin to slow down in about 2 weeks, at which point it is time to take out the scraps. When you remove the cover, you may see a clear film developing on top. It is the beginning of the vinegar mother. Remove it (trying to keep it whole, if possible) and set it aside while you're straining out the fruit solids. Replace the mother and cover the jar.

7. Check the vinegar in a month, when you should have nice acidity. However, it may take another month or two to fully develop. Test the pH: It should be 4.0 or below.

8. Bottle the finished vinegar, saving the mother for another batch or sharing with a friend. Use immediately, or age to allow it to mellow and develop flavors.

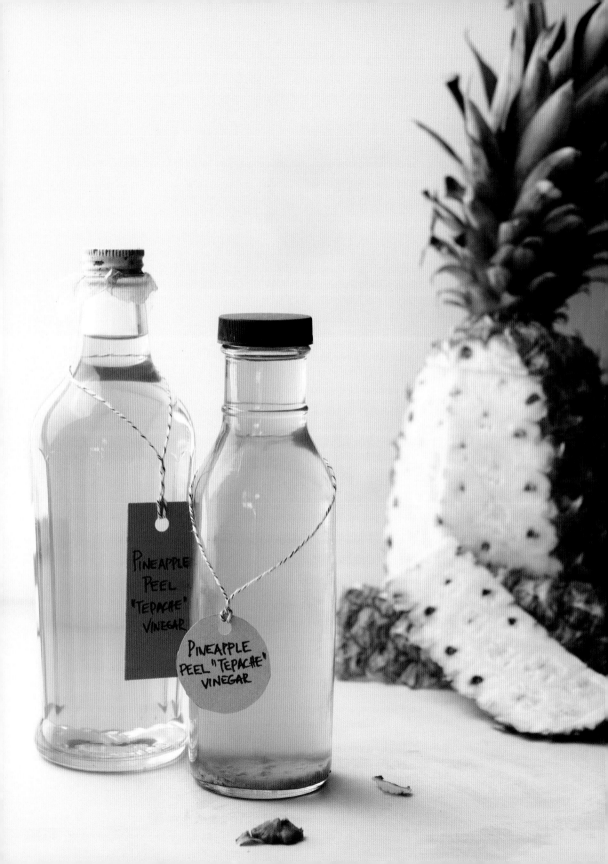

Pineapple Skin and Core Vinegar

HAVE YOUR PINEAPPLE, tepache, and vinegar, too! This recipe epitomizes whole utilization. Eat the pineapple, then ferment the scraps to make tepache: a simple, quick, lightly boozy, funky beverage that's popular in parts of Mexico. Then proceed to make vinegar; this recipe adds an optional second round of sugar to boost the ABV for higher acidity and longer shelf life. The raw vinegar isn't strictly necessary; it's more of an insurance policy than anything.

Because this recipe is ultimately for vinegar, I omit the traditional tepache spices. Should you want to play with different flavors, though, you can add your choice of the following: one cinnamon stick, three or four whole cloves, five or six peppercorns (or a long pepper, if you have it), one star anise, or a teaspoon of coriander seeds. Finally, I love tamarind and found adding a few tamarind pods to the mixture also makes a delicious tepache vinegar.

YIELD about 1½ quarts

Outer peel and core of 1 pineapple

4 tamarind pods (optional)

6–8 cups (1.4–1.9 L) room-temperature unchlorinated water

1¾ cups (350 g) piloncillo (see Note) or turbinado sugar

½ cup (118 mL) raw, unfiltered, unpasteurized vinegar

1. Place the pineapple peels, core, and tamarind pods (if using) in a sanitized half-gallon jar or ceramic vessel.

2. In a bowl, dissolve 1½ cups of the piloncillo in about 2 cups of the warm water. Pour the sugar water over the pineapple, then use some of the remaining water to fill the jar to the rim. Stir everything together.

3. Cover the jar with a piece of unbleached cotton (butter muslin or tightly woven cheesecloth), or a basket-style paper coffee filter. Secure with a string, a rubber band, or a threaded metal canning band. This is to keep out fruit flies.

NOTE: Piloncillo is an unprocessed Mexican brown sugar with a light, smoky molasses flavor.

4. Place on your counter or in another spot that is around 75°F/25°C.

5. Let sit for 3 to 5 days. It will ferment faster in warmer conditions. Taste it on day 3; it is tepache when it has a nice tart, light alcoholic funk. Let it continue

recipe continues on next page

further if it's still sweet; otherwise, pour the tepache through a strainer into a clean jar. (You can drink a glass to your success.)

6. To produce a light vinegar, simply keep the tepache covered with a cloth and let it continue to ferment. For a stronger vinegar, mix the remaining ¼ cup piloncillo sugar with 1 cup water and the raw vinegar. Cover and set in a spot that is 75° to 86°F/25° to 30°C.

7. Check the vinegar in a month, when you should have nice acidity. However, it may take another month or two to fully develop. Test the pH: It should be 4.0 or below.

8. Bottle the finished vinegar, saving the mother for another batch or sharing with a friend. Use immediately, or age to allow it to mellow and develop flavors.

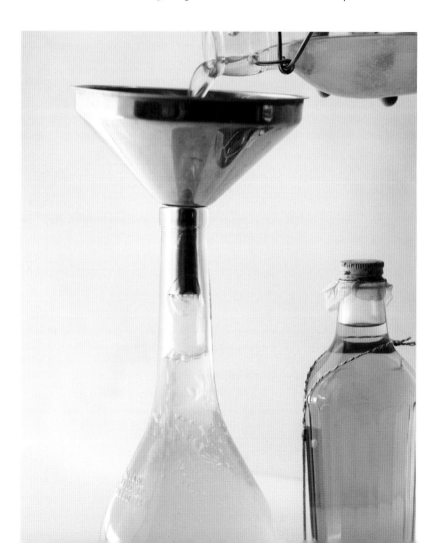

WHOLE UTILIZATION SQUARED

Scrap vinegar poured on scrap bread: In Oaxaca, there is a traditional street snack called *piedrazo*. A piedrazo is stale bread with fruit and vinegar served in a plastic bag with a spoon. Piedrazos are sold in the streets and are quite popular. The vinegar used in piedrazos is made locally by traditional cooks.

VINEGAR STUDY:
VINEGAR FROM RICE AND PASTA WATERS

This vinegar is made not from the rice but from the milky, starchy liquid that remains after soaking rice. This soaking water is said to contain many minerals and vitamins that leached out of the rice. It has been used for centuries in Asia as a (miracle) hair treatment. I decided to use soaking water from white rice to make vinegar, and it was very successful—surprisingly so. It fermented without much care on my part and formed a mother easily. It was not only nicely acidic but it retained sweetness. In short, tasty.

The sugar content is minimal, so this vinegar is made with added sugar. I used granulated white sugar at a rate of 4.4 ounces (125 g) per quart (946 mL) of rice water. I added a crushed Chinese yeast ball to this mixture. The pH was very high, so I didn't want to let the alcohol fermentation go too long. Given the open vessel, the high pH makes it more susceptible to surface yeast. After two days, I added ½ cup (118 mL) raw vinegar per quart. This vinegar took two months to develop a mother and another two to taste done. I began it during the hot temperatures of August, but it mostly aged in cooler-than-ideal (for vinegar) temperatures of my fermentation cave. It was surprisingly citrusy. Upon aging, it retained a residual sweetness that gave it a lemonade flavor. Despite the delicious success, it is not an official recipe because I didn't have a chance to test it multiple times—but I will be making it again.

Forager, chef, and vinegar maker Jitti Chaithiraphant of Heritage Ferments has been making inspired vinegars from myriad base ingredients for many years. He shared a similar idea that I also have only partially tested: Use the water from cooking pasta! He says any kind of pasta works, except egg noodles. Jitti proclaims egg noodle vinegar gross but soba and other pastas delicious. His pro tip is that you can't salt your cooking water if you plan on turning it to vinegar.

Allow the water to cool, then take an SG or Brix measurement (page 56). In my trials, I found Brix to work better, because of the viscosity of pasta water. I found quite a bit of variation in Brix levels, depending on the pasta. Based on your reading, add sugar at a rate of 4.4 ounces (125 g) per quart (946 mL) of pasta water. I also found a Chinese yeast ball (see page 217) to be the most effective type of yeast. And be sure to add the vinegar starter after two days of fermentation to bring down that pH.

Universal Scrap Vinegar

YOU CAN USE ANY fruit scraps you like with this recipe: strawberry hulls that have been topped with a bit of fruit; cherry pits that have gone through pitting but still retain a lot of juicy fruit bits; the mashed steamed skins and such that come from a steam juicer; the mash after running fruit through a food mill; the fiber that comes out of your juicer after making apple, beet, or ginger juice; or tiny, seedy wild rose hips. You get the idea. Besides flavor, the skins and bits of fruit often provide wild yeasts as well as nutrients for any yeast you use. If you are using organic skins and peelings, feel free to omit the added yeast. Like the pomace left from pressing apples, though, scrap vinegar often needs to be fortified with a sugar source.

The amount of scrap material called for in this recipe may seem unattainable at first glance. Don't worry: You can collect and store scraps in the freezer until you have enough. I like to use closer to a pound, but there is a lot of leeway. Use what you can gather, and combine ingredients that seem like they'd be tasty together.

YIELD
about 2 quarts

½–1 pound (225–450 g) fruit/vegetable skins, cores, leftover mash from straining, or basically anything left from a fruit or vegetable project

¾ cup (155 g) sugar, any kind

1½ quarts (1.4 L) unchlorinated water, just off the boil

OPTIONAL:

½ teaspoon (1 g) wine yeast hydrated in ¼ cup (59 mL) unchlorinated water that has been warmed to 104°F/40°C; or ½ cup (118 mL) room-temperature wild yeast starter (page 53)

¾ cup (177 mL) raw, unfiltered, unpasteurized vinegar, or a vinegar mother

1. Combine the fruit and sugar in a sanitized half-gallon jar. Stir in 1 quart of the just-boiled water. Use the remaining water to fill the jar to the neck.

2. Let the mixture cool to room temperature, then add the vinegar and yeast (if using).

3. Stir well with a wooden spoon. You want to get some oxygen in the mix. However, make sure the fruit scraps themselves stay submerged; otherwise they can become a host for undesirable opportunistic bacteria.

4. Cover the jar with a piece of unbleached cotton (butter muslin or tightly woven cheesecloth), or a basket-style paper coffee filter. Secure with a string, a rubber band, or a threaded metal canning band. This is to keep out fruit flies.

5. Place on your counter or in another spot that is 75° to 86°F/25° to 30°C.

6. Stir once a day with a wooden spoon for the first 5 or 6 days, then stir now and then, if you remember. You may see bubbles: That is good.

7. The ferment will begin to slow down in about 2 weeks, at which point it is time to take out the scraps. When you remove the cover, you may see a film developing on top. It is the beginning of the vinegar mother. Remove and set it aside while you're straining out the fruit solids.

8. Transfer the almost-vinegar (and the vinegar mother, if you have one) to a clean jar and cover again.

9. Check the vinegar in a month, when you should have nice acidity. However, it may take another month or two to fully develop. Test the pH: It should be 4.0 or below.

10. Bottle the finished vinegar, saving the mother for another batch or sharing with a friend. Use immediately, or age to allow it to mellow and develop flavors.

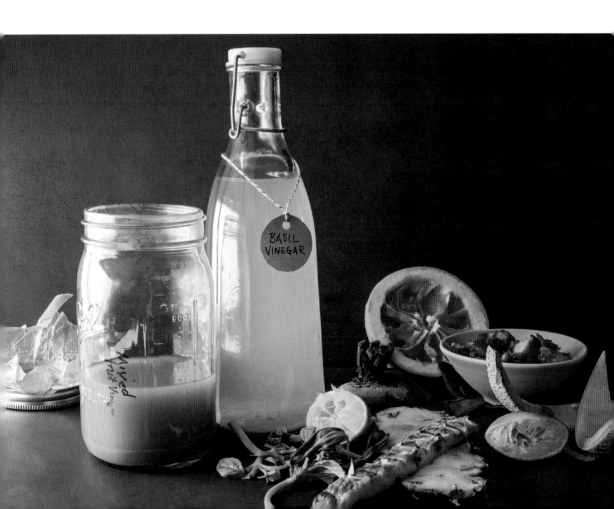

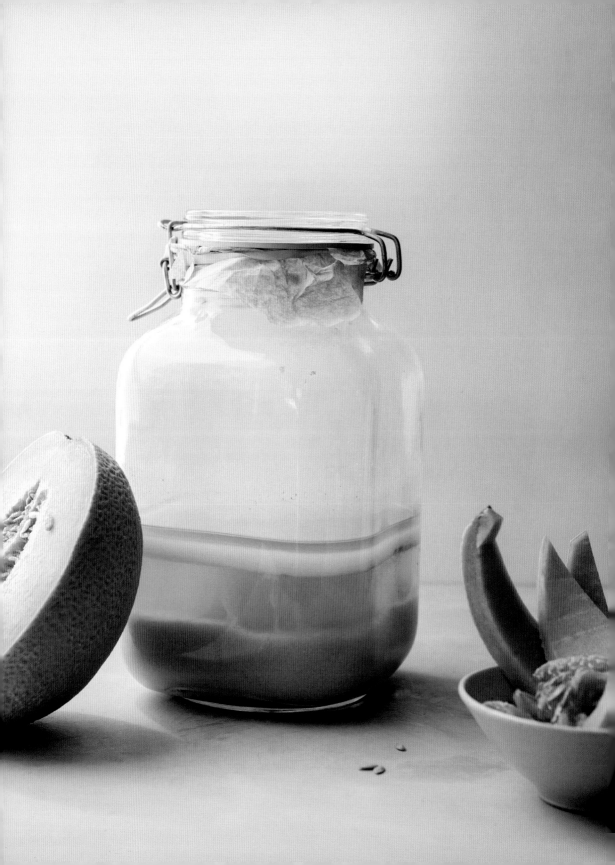

Universal Amazake Scrap Vinegar

THIS VINEGAR IS A koji-based scrap vinegar; the sugar comes from the amazake, and the flavor comes from the fruit scraps. I learned this vinegar-making technique from Chef Jeremy Umansky, co-owner of Larder Delicatessen and Bakery in Cleveland, Ohio, and coauthor of *Koji Alchemy*. Use any fruits or vegetable scraps—melon rinds, mango skins, or other peelings. For the sake of simplicity, this recipe calls for ready-made, rice-based amazake. If you'll be making your own amazake, according to the recipe on page 87, use any grain or starchy vegetable, and add the fruit scraps at the incubation stage.

YIELD
about 1½ quarts

1 pound (450 g) fruit scraps, scrubbed clean

3 cups amazake (690 g)

½ teaspoon (1 g) wine yeast hydrated in ¼ cup (59 mL) unchlorinated water, warmed to 104°F/40°C; or ½ cup (118 mL) room-temperature wild yeast starter (page 53)

1 cup (237 mL) raw, unfiltered, unpasteurized vinegar, with or without the mother

1 quart (0.9 L) room-temperature, unchlorinated water

1. Combine the fruit scraps and amazake in a blender or food processor and purée.

2. Pour the purée into a sanitized gallon jar and add the hydrated yeast liquid or the wild yeast starter. Stir well with a wooden spoon.

3. Cover the jar with a piece of unbleached cotton (butter muslin or tightly woven cheesecloth), or a basket-style paper coffee filter. Secure with a string, a rubber band, or a threaded metal canning band. This is to keep out fruit flies.

4. Let ferment for 48 hours or more—keeping it at room temperature and stirring daily—or until yeast activity (heavy bubbling) has slowed down.

5. Add the raw vinegar.

6. Continue fermentation at room temperature, or 75° to 86°F (25° to 30°C). Stir daily for the first two weeks. At this point you don't need to monitor it very often; just check in on it every few weeks for the next 6 weeks to 2 months, or until the vinegar tastes right. Check the pH: It should be 4.0 or below. If surface yeast begins to form, continue to stir regularly.

7. Strain through a fine-mesh strainer to remove the thicker lees. Leave cloudy, or allow to settle and rack off the clear vinegar.

8. Bottle. Use immediately, or age to allow it to mellow and develop flavors.

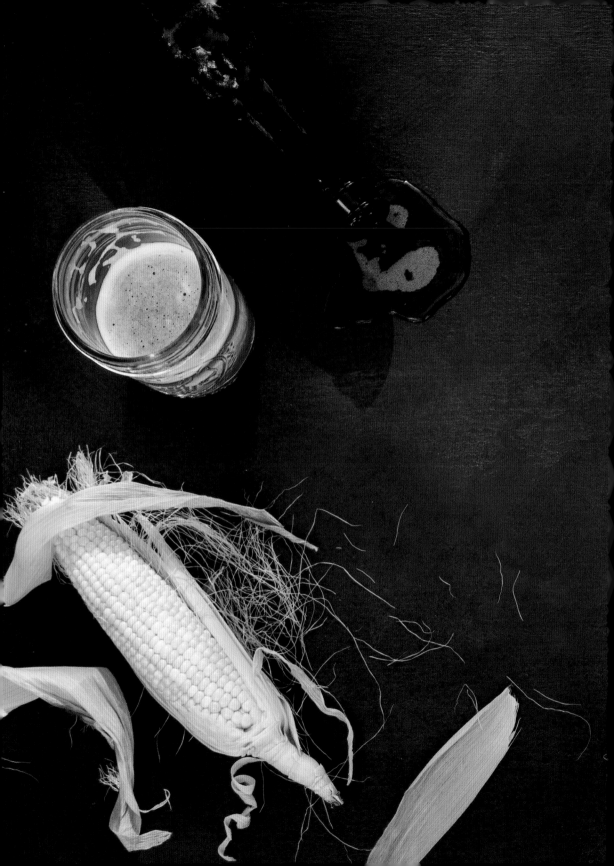

MEET ᴛʜᴇ MAKER

RICHARD STEWART,
MADHOUSE VINEGAR

The MadHouse Vinegar Co. is housed at the historic Carriage House Farm in North Bend, Ohio. Their vinegar is made from sustainably grown ingredients including native plants such as pawpaw, spicebush, and elderberries. However, MadHouse got its start making small-batch vinegars from the waste stream of small-batch beverages produced in the area around Cincinnati—the beer breweries, cider houses, vineyards, and distilleries of southwestern Ohio and northern Kentucky. From spent grains, weak worts (the sugary liquid left over from brewing), and skunked beer to culled wines or ciders: Each of these makers has waste, which used to be poured down the drain or sent to a landfill until MadHouse stepped in.

These days, Richard Stewart and his business partner, Justin Dean, turn these unwanted ingredients into delicious, one-of-a-kind vinegars. Consumers have come to expect (and appreciate) that each batch is unique, but Richard doesn't necessarily see the idea of upcycled, zero-waste vinegar as a key selling point; he thinks most people aren't used to seeing the terms *waste* and *recycled* associated with food products.

The genesis for the vinegar business started with a simple desire to build another brick in the local food system—to create, as Richard says, "vinegar of the region [that] reflects the alcohol of the region." With the availability of beer, Richard and Justin thought that malt vinegar wasn't a difficult reach for people's palates, so they started making vinegar with wort from local breweries. Then the breweries began to offer them beers that were too far gone: beer with its hop flavor breaking down, stouts no longer selling in summer, oxidized beers, and so on. MadHouse started working with a distillery to source aging barrels that were no longer used, then found the same resource at local wineries. Barrels that were done in these businesses were just perfect for theirs.

Suddenly, great inputs were everywhere. Now Richard and Justin produce a mint vinegar from candy canes and vinegar made from unsold sweet corn (the mash is made from the cobs and kernels). Richard talked about rescuing food from supermarkets—such as turning overripe bananas into balsamic-style vinegar—but said, "one company can only do so much."

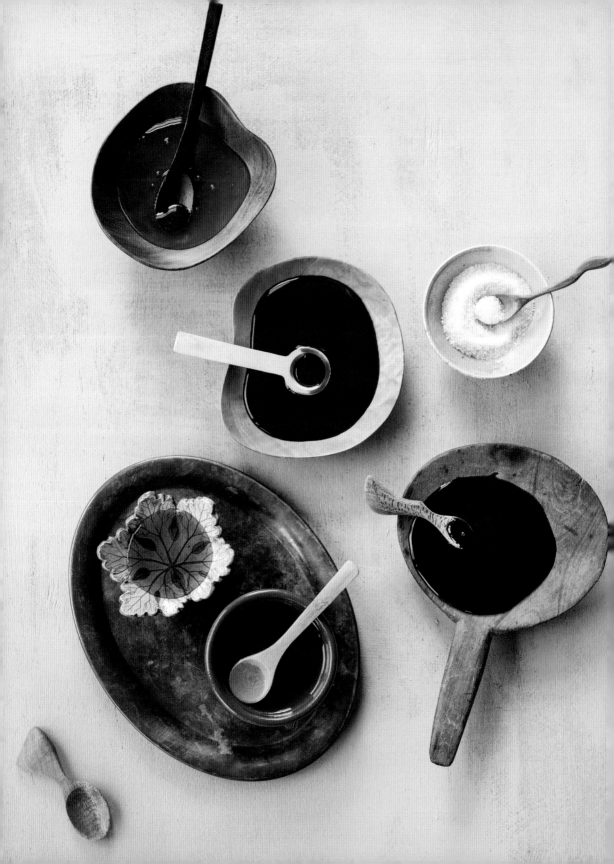

CHAPTER 8

VINEGARS FROM HONEY, SYRUPS, AND JUICES

THESE ARE SUCH EASY VINEGARS, you could almost say, "Just add water." Syrups and juices are a wonderful way to work with flavors when you don't have access to the fresh version of the ingredients—using palm syrup to make coconut vinegar, for example (page 202). I find that using syrups is also quite economical; for example, the cost of making a beautiful reddish date vinegar (page 205) with syrup doesn't even compare to the cost of making it with fresh dates. Your larder can be stocked with unique flavors from honey, maple syrup, molasses, malted barley, date syrup, palm sugar, and agave. Bottled juices from the grocery store fit in this same category of easy-to-access base ingredients that can become delicious, unique vinegars.

Beet Vinegar

BEET VINEGAR IS beautiful and tasty, with a nice acidity that is accompanied by a residual sweetness. The quality of the beets really shines through. This recipe demonstrates how you can make vinegar from bottled pasteurized juice from the grocery store. I like how a little time, intention, and fermentation breathe in life and flavors. Feel free to use this recipe with other bottled juices; I have tried it with pomegranate, cherry, and mango juices with good results.

If you want to use fresh beets, juice them and follow the process in the recipe for Carrot-Ginger Vinegar (page 141). You could also make an amazake vinegar by breaking down cooked beets with rice koji, or just growing the koji directly on the beet, as shown in Purple Sweet Potato Vinegar (page 165).

YIELD
about 1 quart

1 quart (946 mL) bottled beet juice

⅓ cup (114 g) honey

1 cup (237 mL) unchlorinated water, warmed to 100°F/38°C

½ teaspoon (1 g) wine yeast, hydrated in ¼ cup (59 mL) unchlorinated water that has been warmed to 104°F/40°C; or ½ cup (118 mL) room-temperature wild yeast starter (page 53)

¾ cup (177 mL) raw, unfiltered, unpasteurized vinegar, or a vinegar mother

1. Pour the beet juice into a sanitized half-gallon jar.

2. Mix the honey and the 1 cup warm water together in a bowl. When the honey is completely incorporated, add the liquid to the beet juice.

3. Add the hydrated yeast liquid or the room-temperature wild yeast starter to the jar. Stir well with a wooden spoon.

4. Cover the jar with a piece of unbleached cotton (butter muslin or tightly woven cheesecloth), or a basket-style paper coffee filter. Secure with a string, a rubber band, or a threaded metal canning band. This is to keep out fruit flies.

5. Place on your counter. Stir with a wooden spoon once a day for the first 5 or 6 days. You may see bubbles: That is good.

6. After 5 or 6 days, add the raw vinegar. Stir again and replace the cover. Place in a spot that is slightly warmer, ideally 75° to 86°F/25° to 30°C.

7. You can continue to stir daily or just let it do its thing. If you don't stir when you remove the cover, you may see a film developing on top of the vinegar. It is the beginning of the vinegar mother.

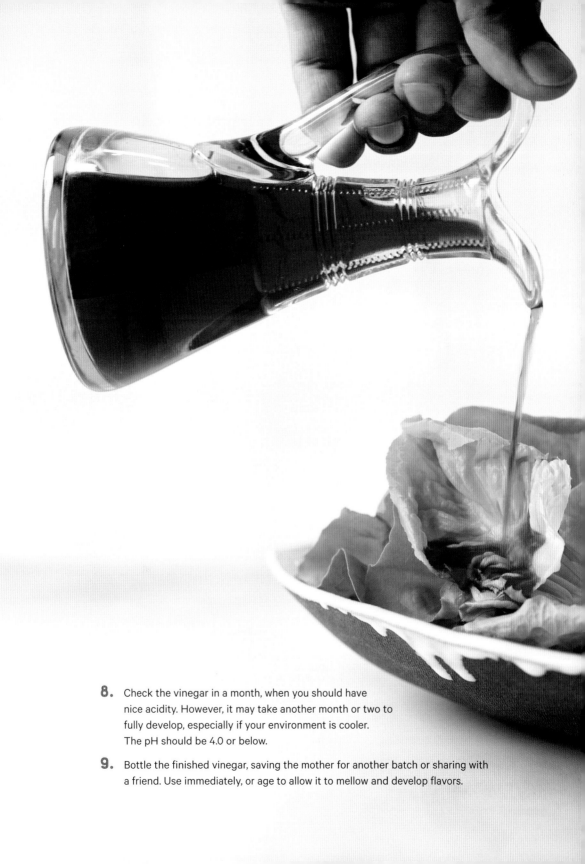

8. Check the vinegar in a month, when you should have nice acidity. However, it may take another month or two to fully develop, especially if your environment is cooler. The pH should be 4.0 or below.

9. Bottle the finished vinegar, saving the mother for another batch or sharing with a friend. Use immediately, or age to allow it to mellow and develop flavors.

Coconut Vinegar

COCONUT VINEGAR is a delicious, mild choice for people who don't love a strong acid flavor. It's traditionally made from the sap of the coconut palm (see Traditional Coconut Vinegar, opposite), often labeled as palm nectar. As such, there is nothing inexpensive about this fermentation (it's more economical than buying coconut vinegar, though). Depending on where you live, the ingredients must be imported but are widely available online or in health foods stores.

What struck me most about this vinegar was that as it aged, the flavor was rich in aminos; it had the umami and underlying richness from the amino acids that you taste in soy sauce. It wasn't until after I'd made a number of batches that I learned that the sap contains 17 amino acids. Additionally, it has vitamin C, B-complex vitamins, a high potassium level, and a low glycemic index. And all this goodness doesn't get lost during fermentation.

**YIELD
about
1½ quarts**

12 ounces (354 g) raw palm nectar

1 quart (946 mL) room-temperature unchlorinated water

½ teaspoon (1 g) wine yeast hydrated in ¼ cup (59 mL) unchlorinated water that has been warmed to 104°F/40°C; or ½ cup (118 mL) room-temperature wild yeast starter (page 53)

2 cups (473 mL) raw, unfiltered, unpasteurized vinegar, or a vinegar mother

1. Pour the palm nectar into a sanitized half-gallon jar. Add the room-temperature water, then stir well with a wooden spoon.

2. Add the hydrated yeast liquid or the room-temperature wild yeast starter to the jar. Stir well with a wooden spoon.

3. Cover the jar with a piece of unbleached cotton (butter muslin or tightly woven cheesecloth), or a basket-style paper coffee filter. Secure with a string, a rubber band, or a threaded metal canning band. This is to keep out fruit flies.

4. Place on your counter or in another spot that is 75° to 86°F/25° to 30°C.

5. Check the vinegar in a month, when you should have nice acidity. However it may take another month or two to fully develop. The pH should be 4.0 or below.

6. Bottle the finished vinegar, saving the mother for another batch or sharing with a friend. Use immediately, or age to allow it to mellow and develop flavors.

Variation:
Coconut Vinegar

YOU CAN SUBSTITUTE coconut water for the palm nectar and water in the recipe on the previous page. Be sure to use the raw pink water, sold under the brand name Harmless Harvest. It is the only one that worked 100 percent of the time for me in the many batches I tested. You will also need to add ⅓ cup (70 g) of coconut sugar (made from the sap) and 1 cup (237 mL) of raw coconut vinegar.

TRADITIONAL COCONUT VINEGAR

Coconut vinegar is traditionally made from the sap of the coconut palm. The blossom stem is snipped at the tip and trained to curve downward into a collection vessel, where the sap drips slowly out. The sap must be collected twice a day; in the warm climate where coconuts grow, it ferments very quickly. Apparently, tapping does no harm to the tree, and one tap can flow for 20 years! This makes it a pretty sustainable product. In the Philippines, this nectar is fermented into a wine called *tubâ* (and where there is wine, there is vinegar). I was introduced to tubâ in Mexico, where it was introduced from the Philippines, by way of Spanish ships in the sixteenth and seventeenth centuries.

TRY THIS: HOT DATE VINEGAR TODDY

This classic hot-toddy cocktail has its roots in palm sap fermentations. The Hindi word *tadi* refers to a beverage made of fermented palm sap. The British defined a hot toddy in 1786 as a "beverage made from alcoholic liquor with hot water, sugar, and spices." Make your favorite hot-toddy recipe, but instead of using lemon, splash in some date syrup vinegar in a nod to fermented palm sap everywhere.

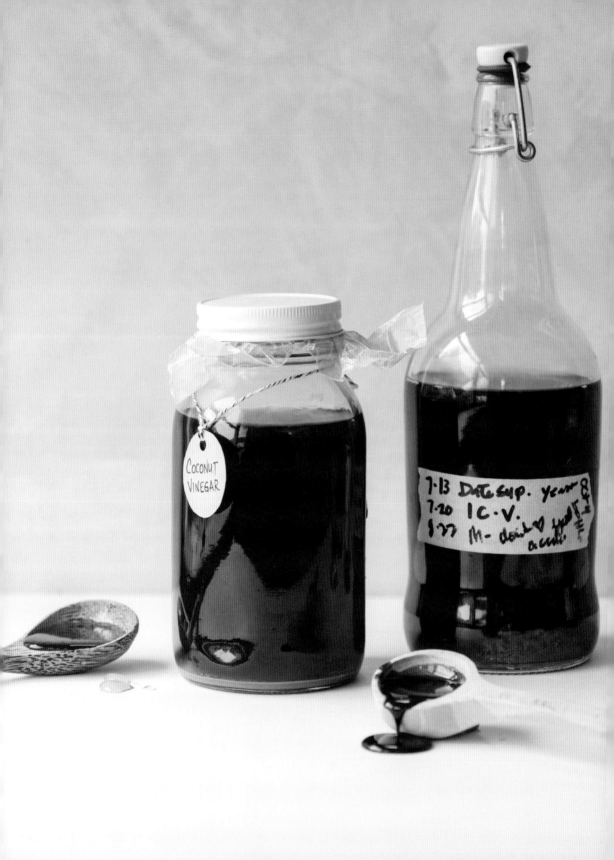

COCONUT
VINEGAR

7·13 Date Syp. Yeas
7·20 1 C · V.
8·27 M· [illegible] good
acidic.

Date Syrup Vinegar

DATE VINEGAR HAILS from lands rich in dates, as you might expect. It also happens to be the first vinegar mentioned in written language: We have evidence that the Babylonians made vinegar from both the fruit and the sap of the date palm. I planned on sharing a recipe using the fruit as well. When it worked I had a thicker, rustic, sweet, wild fermented vinegar. When it didn't, it was not good. My success rate was somewhere around 50 percent—admittedly disappointing. The syrup vinegar never failed with its crisp, clean acidity. Interestingly, as it ages, the amino flavors that I associate with other palm vinegars come forward—in this case, they are much lighter than those of the coconut vinegar. Traditionally, this vinegar is made from the sap of the date palm. The date syrup available in the United States is not concentrated date palm sap but rather the extracted nectar from the dates themselves: Water is added to the dates and then everything is heated, blended, and strained, and the water is set to evaporate. What's left is the date nectar.

YIELD
about 2 quarts

12 ounces (340 g) date syrup

7 cups (1.7 L) unchlorinated water, warmed to 85°F/29°C

½ teaspoon (1 g) wine yeast hydrated in ¼ cup (59 mL) unchlorinated water that has been warmed to 104°F/40°C; or ½ cup (118 mL) room-temperature wild yeast starter (page 53)

1 cup (237 mL) raw, unfiltered, unpasteurized vinegar, or a vinegar mother

1. Combine the syrup and the 7 cups water in a sanitized half-gallon jar. Stir well with a wooden spoon.

2. Add the hydrated yeast liquid or the room temperature wild yeast starter to the jar. Stir well with a wooden spoon.

3. Cover the jar with a piece of unbleached cotton (butter muslin or tightly woven cheesecloth), or a basket-style paper coffee filter. Secure with a string, a rubber band, or a threaded metal canning band. This is to keep out fruit flies.

4. Place on your counter or in another spot that is 75° to 86°F/25° to 30°C.

5. Check the vinegar in 6 weeks, when you should have nice acidity. The alcohol develops quickly. In my experience, it isn't particularly tasty early on and is slightly bitter. It may take another month or two to fully develop flavors.

6. Bottle the finished vinegar, saving the mother for another batch or sharing with a friend. Use immediately, or age to allow it to mellow and develop flavors.

Mead to Honey Vinegar

HONEY VINEGAR STARTS with honey wine—which most people know as mead. Honey is chock-full of complex sugars, but as rich as honey is, it often doesn't have enough essential nutrients to see the yeast through its job of gobbling up all the sugar and converting it to alcohol. For this reason when making your first few batches, Jennifer Holmes (a beekeeper in Stuart, Florida; see page 208), recommends adding fruit that contains both more sugar, nutrients, and natural yeast (if it's organic and unwashed). To keep those yeasts well fed and give a nice edge to a successful batch of mead, use spring or filtered water, not distilled.

I was not able to successfully short-cut the process with a simultaneous ferment. I found that the mead needed to fully ferment and develop before I could make honey vinegar. Jennifer Holmes shared her mead-making process for this recipe; you can make it with either mead yeast (see Notes on opposite page) or a wild starter. If you would like to start with purchased mead rather than making your own, you'll need four 750 mL bottles. The vinegar-making process begins at step 5. This recipe also includes an optional, final honey sweetening step for a full-bodied, rich, sweet vinegar.

YIELD
1 gallon

3 quarts (2.8 L) unchlorinated water, warmed to around 100°F/38°C

3 pounds (1.36 kg) honey, plus more for back-sweetening

1 tablespoon (15 mL) lemon or lime juice

1 cup (240 g) foraged or local fruit, large fruit chopped or puréed; small fruit pulsed in a food processor (optional; see Notes)

1 tablespoon (15 g) dried herbs, or 3 tablespoons (45 g) fresh herbs or spices (optional; see Notes)

1 tablespoon (15 g) commercial mead yeast hydrated in ¼ cup (59 mL) unchlorinated water, warmed to 104°F/40°C; or ½ cup (118 mL) room-temperature wild yeast starter (page 53)

1 cup (237 mL) raw, unfiltered, unpasteurized vinegar, with or without the mother

1. Combine the warm water and honey in a sanitized 2-gallon stainless-steel stock pot or food-grade bucket until blended. Add the lemon juice and the fruit and herbs or spices, if using. Stir vigorously to mix and aerate. Adding oxygen at this stage and through the next 12 to 24 hours enlivens and feeds the yeasts present and introduces more yeast from the environment.

2. Cover the pot with a cloth, secured with a string or rubber band to keep out fruit flies. Stir any time you think of it in the next 12 to 24 hours. You may see some bubbling or foam develop on the surface; that is fine.

3. After 24 hours, add the hydrated yeast or the room-temperature wild yeast starter. Stir well with a wooden spoon and cover again with the cloth.

4. Ferment for about 2 weeks, or until you see the fermentation slow down.

5. At this point you will want to get the liquid off the fruit pulp solids and the crashed yeast sediment at the bottom of the pot. You can either use tubing to rack the liquid into a sanitized 1-gallon jar, or pour it carefully through a fine sieve, stopping once you reach the lees.

6. Cover the jar with a piece of unbleached cotton (butter muslin or tightly woven cheesecloth), or a basket-style paper coffee filter. Secure with a string, a rubber band, or a threaded metal canning band.

7. Check the vinegar in a month, when you should have nice acidity. However, it may take another month or two to fully develop. Bottle the vinegar, saving the mother for another batch or sharing with a friend.

Optional final steps for a back-sweetened honey-sweet honey vinegar

8. Pasteurize the honey vinegar according to the instructions on page 106.

9. For every cup (237 mL) of cooled, pasteurized vinegar, mix in 2 to 4 tablespoons (30 to 60 g) of liquid honey, carefully warmed to 100°F (78°C). If you prefer a richer, sweeter vinegar, add more honey. (I have found that more than 4 tablespoons [60 mL] per cup [237 mL] makes the vinegar too sweet for my taste.)

10. Bottle the finished vinegar in airtight bottles. It will last indefinitely with no air contact.

NOTES: Here are some nomenclature fun facts: When you add fruit, you are making a melomel; with spices and fruit, it becomes a metheglin. And when you make it with apple juice, it is a cyser.

Mead yeast Lavlin ICV-D47 is a tolerant and widely used commercial yeast for making a dry or semi-dry mead.

If you'd like to produce a drinkable mead—so that you can enjoy some as a beverage and turn some into vinegar—use a sanitized brewing bucket and airlock lid for steps 1–4.

THE IMPORTANCE
OF SOURCE

Just as you want to use good, organic produce for your fruit- and vegetable-based vinegars, it's important to find a sustainable source of honey if you're going to make mead to turn into honey vinegar. With the increasing use of chemical agents on the crops bees forage from, it's more important than ever to source honey from sustainable, small-scale producers. This isn't just for the sake of the bees (which is important!) but also because the way in which forage crops are grown and treated ultimately affects the flavor of the honey.

Jennifer Holmes, a beekeeper and honey sommelier-in-training from Stuart, Florida (whose recipe for mead appears on page 206), has developed a reverence for honey over the course of her career, as well as an understanding of how environmental factors affect the health of bees and the flavor of their honey. For example, when the citrus industry was in rapid decline in Florida because of widespread disease, very few trees were producing nectar and the use of chemicals was at an all-time high. The first thing Jennifer noticed was that she could no longer smell the heady orange blossom perfume that usually filled the air. She didn't think the bees would produce much honey during the bloom— and they didn't. The honey produced that year was dark and flavorless, and there was very little of it.

Jennifer's training as a honey sommelier— which, essentially, means learning how to identify honey by taste and smell—means that she can detect unique flavors and markers but also chemicals, smoke, (unintended) fermentation, or adulteration (added sugar or syrup) in honey. She guesses that with the lack of forage and difficulties facing pollinators worldwide as they are assaulted by everything from chemicals on crops to mites and unknown factors, honey in its natural state will become more and more rare in the coming years if we do not make drastic changes. What may be available will be adulterated and lack the fine qualities, aromas, flavor profiles, and health benefits.

Using local honey is a way to support your small local beekeepers who are mindful of their practices and working with organic producers to grow healthy crops for the bees to forage from. Using quality ingredients will make your final products amazing.

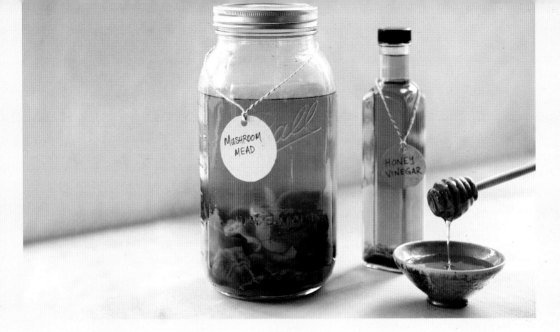

OLD-TIME HONEY VINEGAR

A 1935 Michigan State College Extension Bulletin by Frederick W. Fabian, titled *Honey Vinegar*, is a quick, fascinating read and offers insight into past efforts to make a value-added product from "honey which would otherwise be lost." Fabian suggests using honey from hives infected with "foul-brood, honey-dew honey, coniferous honey, honey from brood combs, washings from the extractor, etc." In order to do this, a great deal of boiling takes place to sterilize the honey, which we now know is not good for the honey or us (see page 270).

The other thing that caught my attention in reading the bulletin is that honey, once diluted (which it must be to ferment), does not have enough nutrients for the yeasts to thrive. This is common knowledge among mead makers, and you often see recipes that add yeast nutrient, raisins, or citrus. Fabian proposes that excellent results have come from chemicals, but since they are not easily obtained (or really used much these days), apple cider can be used to feed a slow mead fermentation, because it has good acid and the minerals needed to feed the yeast. This seems like a nice combination of a mead and cyser (honey cider) to

me. But his formula indicates a much higher ratio of honey to liquid than any mead or cyser recipe I have seen.

His Formula No. 3 calls for 30 to 35 gallons of liquid honey, 7 to 8 gallons of cider, and 18 to 22 gallons of water. This is boiled for 10 minutes and placed in a clean barrel with *Saccharomyces ellipsoideus*, a wine yeast, which he notes will produce an alcohol with 14 percent ABV or higher.

My favorite part, though, is his discussion of the mother. "The vinegar bacteria form a smooth, more or less glistening film on the surface of the honey solution. This film is commonly known as 'mother of vinegar' *and should never be disturbed under any circumstances*. It is customary to float the film on clean beech shavings to prevent it from sinking. . . . Once the film has sunken, it takes several weeks for a new film to form. This greatly increases the time to make vinegar. . . ." We now know that the cellulose formed is not integral to the production of vinegar. But in 1935, microbiology was still relatively new. He goes on to say, "Furthermore when the film sinks, other bacteria are likely to decompose it and produce substances of disagreeable tastes and odors."

Earthy Umami Cyser to Vinegar

CYSER (HONEY CIDER) MAKES an excellent, special apple cider vinegar. This particular cyser was inspired by a savory, garlic-mushroom mead recipe from Jereme Zimmerman, author of *Make Mead Like a Viking*, which I actually made with no garlic and more mushrooms than the recipe called for. Christopher can attest to the pleasure sounds that issued forth as I tasted the mead's umami. I admit, I was torn about turning it into vinegar, as was my original intention, so I did half the batch. The mushroom notes were delightful, and I experimented further, using other mushrooms.

I use dried shiitake, dried reishi, and dried turkey tails because they are easy to source. I have also used lion's mane and oyster mushrooms found in our forest. Use any wildcrafted ingredients you can find; just be 100 percent certain of their identity before you use them. Also, it is a good practice to cook your mushrooms before using. One way is to steam them for 20 minutes or so. Another way is to dehydrate them at a high temperature (above 160°F/71°C) before using them for fermentation; I find this method improves the flavor and quality of the fermentation.

YIELD
1 gallon

1½ cups (50–55 g) loosely packed roughly chopped dried shiitake, turkey tail, and reishi mushrooms, in equal amounts

1 cup (237 mL) unchlorinated water, just off the boil

1⅓ cups (308 mL) quality honey

10 raisins

3 quarts (2.8 L) unpasteurized apple juice

1 teaspoon (1 g) mead yeast: Lalvin ICV-71B or ICV-D47, hydrated in ¼ cup (59 mL) unchlorinated water, warmed to 104°F/40°C

¼–¾ cup (59–177 mL) raw, unfiltered, unpasteurized vinegar, or a vinegar mother

1. Reconstitute the mushrooms in the boiling water in a medium bowl.

2. When the water cools to 100°F/38°C, remove the mushrooms and set them aside. Measure ⅔ cup (160 mL) of the soaking liquid and mix that with the honey in another bowl. Stir until the honey is dissolved.

3. Pour the honey mixture into a sanitized 1-gallon jar or jug. Add the mushrooms and raisins. Pour in enough of the apple juice to fill within 2 to 3 inches of the top. Stir to combine the juice and honey mixture.

4. Add the hydrated yeast liquid to the jar. Stir well with a wooden spoon.

5. Cover the jar with a piece of unbleached cotton (butter muslin or tightly woven cheesecloth), or a basket-style paper coffee filter. Secure with a string, a rubber band, or a threaded metal canning band. This is to keep out fruit flies.

6. Let the vessel sit for a few weeks to a month in a spot that is 55° to 65°F/13° to 18°C.

7. The primary fermentation is finished when half to three-quarters of the sugars have been consumed, which you can determine by noting that no bubbles are being produced.

8. At this point, if the jar has been open to oxygen, acetic bacteria are already present, and you will want to keep it all going toward vinegar. However, if not, use food-safe tubing to rack any cyser you want to keep as cyser into sanitized bottles. Cap and put them in a cabinet to age. Transfer the rest to a new clean jar, straining out the mushrooms.

9. You can cover the new jar with the cover from step 5 and leave as is; bacteria will move in. Or add ¼ cup raw vinegar for every quart (946 mL) of cyser you are fermenting to vinegar.

10. Place on your counter or in another spot that is 75° to 86°F/25° to 30°C.

11. Check the vinegar in a month, when you should have nice acidity. However, it may take another month or two to fully develop.

12. Bottle the finished vinegar, saving the mother for another batch or sharing with a friend. Use immediately, or age to allow it to mellow and develop flavors.

Maple Syrup Vinegar

MAPLE SYRUP VINEGAR IS LOVELY. It has a great acidity and a little residual sweetness. The longest I have had any age at the writing of this book is 6 months; it is smooth, but to my tastes does not have distinctive maple syrup notes. Maple syrup is a good sugar source in that it is high in sugar content, so a little goes a long way. It takes 5 cups of water to bring the ABV to the 1.060 range, which will put the final acidity into the right range. The pH also begins on the acidic side, which makes this less susceptible to early surface yeast growth. This is why the vinegar is added quite soon in the fermentation.

YIELD
1½ quarts

1½ cups (420 g) maple syrup

7½ cups (1.8 L) unchlorinated water, warmed to 85°F/29°C

½ teaspoon (1 g) wine yeast hydrated in ¼ cup (59 mL) unchlorinated water that has been warmed to 104°F/40°C, or ½ cup (118 mL) room-temperature wild yeast starter (page 53)

1½ cups (355 mL) raw, unfiltered, unpasteurized vinegar, or a vinegar mother

1. Combine the maple syrup and the warm water in a sanitized half-gallon jar. Stir well with a wooden spoon.

2. Add the hydrated yeast liquid or the room-temperature wild yeast starter to the jar. Stir well with a wooden spoon.

3. Cover the jar with a piece of unbleached cotton (butter muslin or tightly woven cheesecloth), or a basket-style paper coffee filter. Secure with a string, a rubber band, or a threaded metal canning band. This is to keep out fruit flies.

4. Place on your counter for 4 days to give the yeast a head start.

5. Add the vinegar (with the mother, if available). Replace the cover and place the jar in a spot that is 75° to 86°F/25° to 30°C.

6. Check the vinegar in a month, when you should have nice acidity. However, it may take another month or two to fully develop. The pH should be 4.0 or below.

7. Bottle the finished vinegar, saving the mother for another batch or sharing with a friend. Use immediately, or age to allow it to mellow and develop flavors.

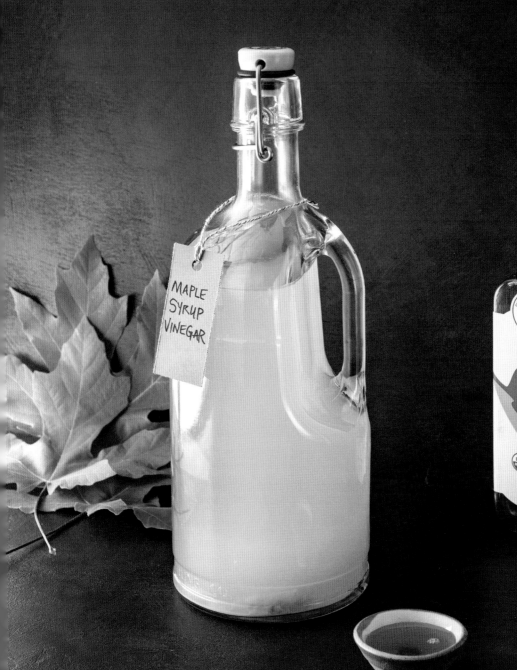

Molasses Vinegar

IF VINEGAR WERE A DARK and stormy night, I think it would be molasses vinegar. It is dark, a little sultry, and definitely does not hide the fact that it is vinegar made from molasses. I find molasses vinegar to be a perfect match for recipes that come from Colonial America; I've added a little to both pumpkin and shoofly pies and in baked beans. My favorite use is as a warm afternoon "tea" or toddy (see Molasses Tea, opposite).

There are different grades of molasses. Unsulfured molasses doesn't mean sulfur has been removed from the product. It means it is processed without adding sulfur dioxide to kill unwanted microbes and combat oxidation (which darkens it). This practice is becoming less common. Molasses can be light, dark, or blackstrap (according to how many times the cane or beet juice is boiled and sugar crystals removed). Blackstrap, which has been boiled three times, can be bitter and has the lowest sugar content—about 45 percent (compared to approximately 70 percent found in dark molasses). If you use blackstrap molasses in the recipe below, use 7 ounces (205 grams). You can also use this recipe with sugar cane syrup to make sugar cane vinegar.

YIELD
about
1½ quarts

½ cup (205 g) dark unsulfured molasses

1 quart (946 mL) room-temperature unchlorinated water

½ teaspoon (1 g) wine yeast hydrated in ¼ cup (59 mL) unchlorinated water that has been warmed to 104°F/40°C; or ½ cup (118 mL) room-temperature wild yeast starter (page 53)

1½ cups (355 mL) raw, unfiltered, unpasteurized vinegar, or a vinegar mother

1. Combine the molasses and the water in a large pot. Warm gently and stir over low heat until the molasses has mixed in. Pour into a sanitized half-gallon jar. Cool to around 100°F/38°C.

2. Add the hydrated yeast liquid or the room-temperature wild yeast starter to the jar. Stir well with a wooden spoon.

3. Cover the jar with a piece of unbleached cotton (butter muslin or tightly woven cheesecloth), or a basket-style paper coffee filter. Secure with a string, a rubber band, or a threaded metal canning band. This is to keep out fruit flies.

4. Place on your counter for 7 days. It will bubble nicely.

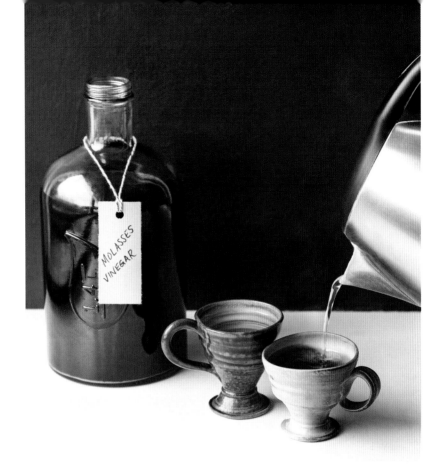

5. On day 7, add the vinegar. Stir well and replace the cover. Place in a spot that is 75° to 86°F/25° to 30°C.

6. Check the vinegar in a month, when you should have nice acidity. However, it may take another month or two to fully develop. Test the pH: It should be 4.0 or below.

7. Bottle the finished vinegar. Use immediately, or age to allow it to mellow and develop flavors.

TRY THIS: MOLASSES TEA

A tablespoon of molasses in a cup of hot water is an alternative to other warm drinks when you need a little something rich that doesn't have caffeine. Blackstrap molasses, in particular, is touted for its high concentration of minerals. Try adding a tablespoon or two of molasses vinegar to this cuppa; the acidity brightens it up.

Rice Vinegar from Brown Rice Syrup

THIS MAKES A DELICIOUS lightly sweet vinegar. The important thing about this recipe is to get a Chinese yeast ball, also called a Shanghai yeast ball or *jing bau* (see A Yeast Ball with a Long History, opposite), which you can find at Asian markets or online. They are inexpensive and work beautifully in this application (whereas my vinegar attempts using wine yeast failed miserably). You will notice there is no vinegar starter. This vinegar takes quite a few months, but it turns nicely and develops a mother on its own (as any working vinegar will eventually do).

YIELD
about
2½ quarts

1 (21-ounce/595 g) jar brown rice syrup

10 cups (2.4 L) unchlorinated water, warmed to 85°F/29°C

1 Chinese yeast ball

¼ cup (59 mL) unchlorinated water, warmed to 104°F/40°C

1. Combine the syrup and the 10 cups warm water in a sanitized gallon jar or other fermentation vessel. Stir well with a wooden spoon until the syrup is completely dissolved.

2. Crush the yeast ball in a mortar and pestle or place in a plastic bag and roll to smash with a rolling pin. Hydrate the yeast by sprinkling it over the ¼ cup warm water. Stir gently, let it sit for 20 minutes, then add the hydrated yeast liquid to the jar and stir well.

3. Cover the jar with a piece of unbleached cotton (butter muslin or tightly woven cheesecloth), or a basket-style paper coffee filter. Secure with a string, a rubber band, or a threaded metal canning band. This is to keep out fruit flies.

4. Place on your counter or in another spot that is 75° to 86°F/25° to 30°C.

5. Check the vinegar in a month, when you should have nice acidity. However, it may take another month or two to fully develop. Test the pH: It should be 4.0 or below.

6. Bottle the finished vinegar, saving the mother for another batch or sharing with a friend. Use immediately, or age to allow it to mellow and develop flavors.

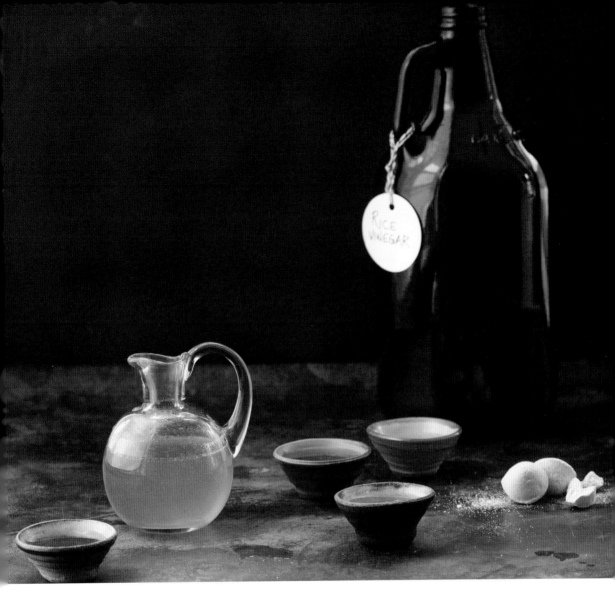

A YEAST BALL WITH A LONG HISTORY

Qu (pronounced *choo*) is the Chinese starter that turns grains into alcohol and then vinegar. These balls are from ancient combinations of fungi, yeasts, and bacteria. Each maker in each region had *qu* that was microbially based in place. For example, some contain herbs that also become part of the final vinegar; others contain fungi that turn the vinegar red. The common yeast balls readily available in Asian markets and online contain a combination of koji (*Aspergillus oryzae*; see page 277) and *Rhizopus oryzae* (commonly used in tempeh), the yeast *Saccharomycopsis fibuligera*, and many types of bacteria. You can use these yeast balls with steamed grains in the same way you would koji rice to saccharify the starches in the grains for fermentation to produce an alcohol from the mash. This becomes your vinegar base.

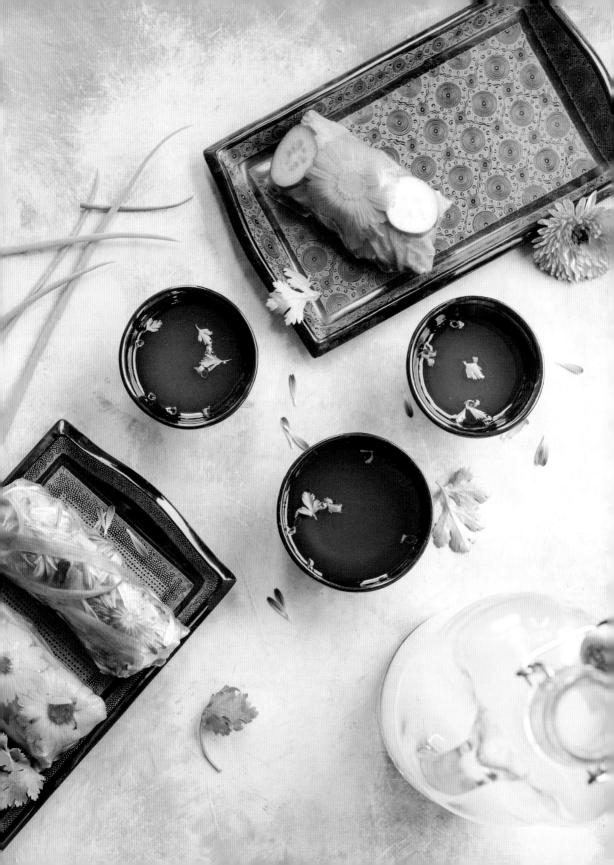

Rice Vinegar from Amazake

RICE VINEGAR BEGINS as amazake that will continue on to ferment into alcohol (sake or doburoku) then, ultimately, vinegar. You can use the amazake at this sweet stage, or at least filch a cup or two. Its next step is a rustic farmhouse ferment, doburoku; again, feel free to drink a little before you take it on to step 4, vinegar. If you drank it all as amazake and doburoku, well, just try again. You will find a similar recipe in Purple Sweet Potato Vinegar (page 165). If you want to use starchy vegetables for your amazake, follow that process. Also feel free to use this recipe and process to experiment with other types of grain.

YIELD
about 1 gallon

3 cups (585 g) purchased brown or white rice koji, or homegrown koji (page 277)

6 cups (1200 g) cooked rice or other grains

6 cups (1.4 L) unchlorinated water, warmed to 135°F/57°C

½ teaspoon (1 g) sake yeast, wine yeast, or bread yeast

¼ teaspoon (1 g) lactic acid for brewing or citric acid, or 1 tablespoon (15 g) lemon juice

6 cups (1.4 L) cool, unchlorinated water

2 cups (473 mL) raw, unfiltered, unpasteurized vinegar

1. Combine the koji and the cooked rice in a sanitized crock or gallon jar. Add the 6 cups warm water. Use a handheld blender to make the mixture as smooth as possible and to increase the surface area of the starches.

2. Set the vessel in your incubation chamber at a temperature between 135° and 138°F/57° and 59°C. Incubate the mixture for 6 to 10 hours or until it has a floral aroma and a mild, sweet taste. (The cooler the incubation, the longer it will take. Also, fresh koji will take less time than dry koji.) Stir the mixture after the first hour and again once or twice during incubation. If you want it sweeter and a little more liquidy, let it ferment a little longer. It will continue to sweeten, but only up to a point. When it hits its limit, the flavor will start to turn slightly sour and have some bitter or alcoholic notes.

3. Add the yeast and lactic acid to the amazake. Let it ferment for 48 hours or more, keeping it between 50°F and 65°F/10°C and 18°C. Temperature is less important if your goal is vinegar, but if you want to enjoy some or all as doburoku, keep it cool—you can even refrigerate it during fermentation.

recipe continues on next page

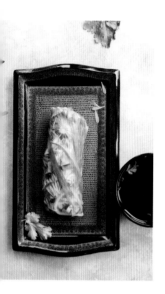

4. After 48 hours of fermentation, what rises to the top of the grain and water mixture will be fairly clear sake. The grain should all be pretty mushy, and there shouldn't be a whole lot of yeast activity—no crackling or heavy bubbling. This stage is still sweet and is when you might want to drink it. As it continues to ferment, it will become more alcoholic and less sweet, which is fine if it is headed to vinegar.

5. Combine the sake you've fermented in step 4 with 6 cups cool water and the vinegar.

6. Transfer to a clean crock or other open fermentation vessel.

7. Cover the jar with a piece of unbleached cotton (butter muslin or tightly woven cheesecloth), or a basket-style paper coffee filter. Secure with a string, a rubber band, or a threaded metal canning band. Let it ferment at room temperature, or 75° to 86°F/25° to 30°C, if possible. Stir daily for the first 2 weeks. Then continue the fermentation for 6 weeks to 2 months, or until the vinegar tastes right. The pH should be 4.0 or below.

8. Bottle the finished vinegar. Use immediately, or allow to age to develop mellow complexity.

CHOOSE YOUR AMAZAKE STARCH

Traditional Japanese amazake is made from rice. However, the process is perfect for making a simple alcohol with koji grown on any grain—corn, millet, barley, oats, you get the idea. Although most vinegars are made from a single type of grain, Korean *ogok* vinegar uses rice and five other grains and the saccharification is done by making a rice starter called *nuruk*. It is then aged in buried clay *onggi* pots. Legumes offer another possibility; Chinese black bean vinegar, which is aged for nine years, is a venerable example of this.

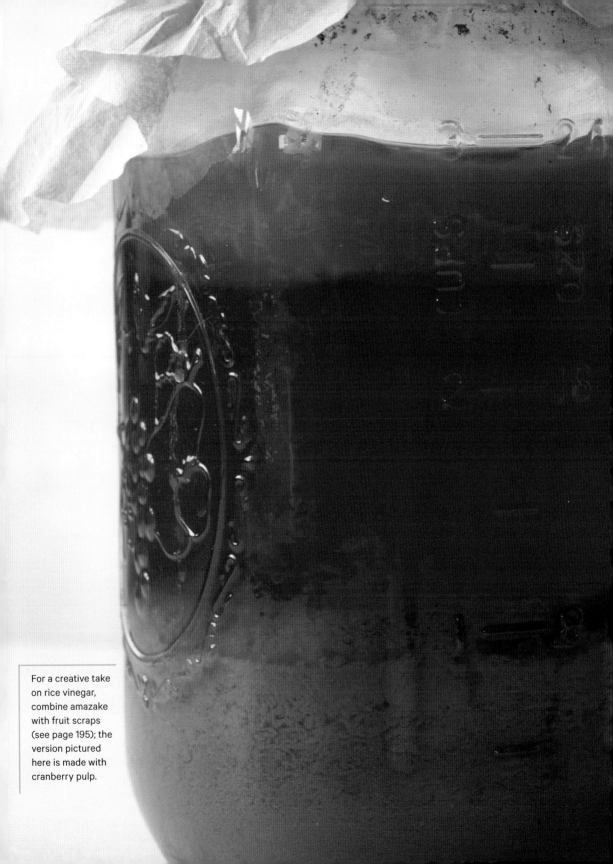

For a creative take on rice vinegar, combine amazake with fruit scraps (see page 195); the version pictured here is made with cranberry pulp.

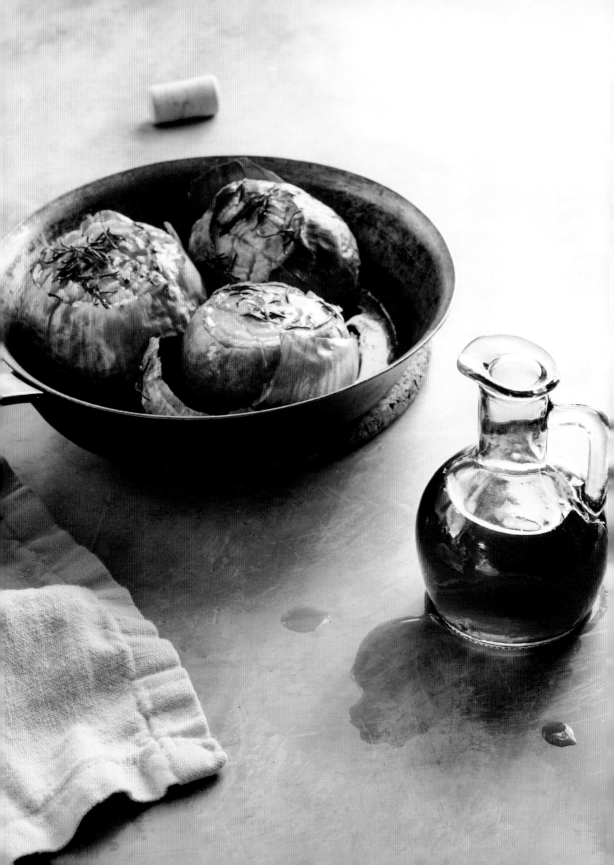

Malt Vinegar

BEFORE THERE WAS CORN SYRUP, food processors and bakers used malted sweeteners. They are stable and contain amino acids, vitamins, minerals, and about 6 percent protein because they are made from whole, sprouted grains. Malting is a saccharification process that involves sprouting and toasting the grains (see More about Malt, page 225). It achieves the same access to the simple sugars that koji does and has been used in Western cultures for thousands of years. You can find traditional malted barley syrup in health food stores and many malted grain extracts at brewer supply stores. This recipe is based on a syrup that is 8 grams of sugar per tablespoon; in my experience, the sugar content in the malt varies wildly. Be sure to check the sugar content listed on the label of your malt syrup, or take a SG or Brix measurement and adjust, as needed, with more or less water.

In this recipe, like in many of these vinegar recipes, you are only brewing to the point of a partial beer, really. In other words, you aren't brewing a beverage you would necessarily drink; you are inviting the yeast to get the party started, so that the acetic bacteria can have theirs. This recipe uses malted barley syrup or another malted grain extract, but if you're a beer brewer and want to start from the beginning, use milled malted barley and make a wort preparation to ferment (which is beyond the scope of this book).

YIELD
about
1½ quarts

- 1 cup (236 g) malted barley syrup, barley malt extract, or other malted grain extract
- 1 quart (0.9 L) room-temperature unchlorinated water
- ½ teaspoon (1 g) wine yeast hydrated in ¼ cup (59 mL) unchlorinated water that has been warmed to 104°F/40°C; or ½ cup (118 mL) room-temperature wild yeast starter (page 53)
- 1½ cups (355 mL) raw, unfiltered, unpasteurized vinegar, or a vinegar mother
- 1–2 tablespoons (15–30 g) barley malt extract

1. Combine the malt and the water in a large pot. Warm gently and stir over medium heat until the malt is mixed in. Pour into a sanitized half-gallon jar. Cool to around 100°F/38°C.

2. Add the hydrated yeast liquid or wild yeast starter to the jar. Stir well with a wooden spoon.

recipe continues on next page

3. Cover the jar with a piece of unbleached cotton (butter muslin or tightly woven cheesecloth), or a basket-style paper coffee filter. Secure with a string, a rubber band, or a threaded metal canning band. This is to keep out fruit flies.

4. Place on your counter for 7 days. It will bubble nicely.

5. On day 7, add the vinegar. Stir well and replace the cover. Place in a spot that is 75° to 86°F/25° to 30°C.

6. Check the vinegar in a month, when you should have nice acidity. However, it may take another month or two to fully develop. Test the pH: It should be 4.0 or below.

7. Back-sweeten with 1 tablespoon of the barley malt extract, or more to taste.

8. Bottle the finished vinegar. Use immediately, or age to allow it to mellow and develop flavors.

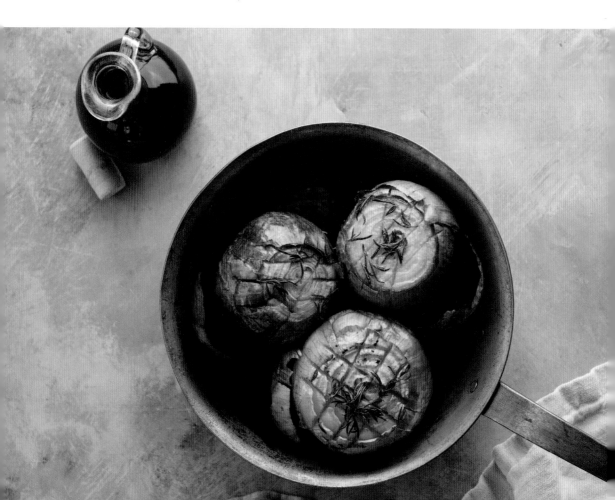

MORE ABOUT MALT

Malting is the process of sprouting and roasting whole grains (most commonly barley), to release the sugars, enzymes, proteins, minerals, amino acids, and flavors to give a brewer his or her raw material. First, the grains are steeped in water to increase their moisture content. Instead of one long soak, the grains are immersed and then pulled out to rest in the air; this is repeated over a few days. The grain begins to germinate, and over the next few days, the grain is kept at a constant temperature and level of airflow, with some type of agitation or movement to keep the developing rootlets from matting up. During this process, enzymes are turning the starches into fermentable sugars. Next, these sprouted grains are dried, a process called kilning. This is where airflow and temperature are manipulated to achieve different colors and flavors. At the end, the rootlets are removed. Finally, the grains are roasted at high temperatures to develop the flavor compounds needed for brewing beer.

Just as wine vinegar, apple cider vinegar, and rice vinegar emerged in regions where wine, cider, and sake were made, malt vinegars developed in places where beer was consumed. The ancient Egyptians were brewing beer around 4000 BCE, so this vinegar has been around a while. That said, what is known as malt vinegar doesn't necessarily start as a beer-based vinegar. As such, there are really two paths to a malted vinegar from any beer, which I will refer to as beer vinegar and malt vinegar.

The biggest difference is that malt vinegar goes straight from a malt wort (malt extract) to fully fermented alcohol and is then acidified, but a beer vinegar becomes beer first. In the typical beer-brewing process, after the wort is made, it is boiled with hops, at least in most cases. This depends, of course, on the beer. Malt vinegar is a little sweeter as it often has either malted syrup or, in cheaper versions, caramel coloring and sweetener added. A porter or a stout beer will give you that malt vinegar flavor and are worth making, but they won't be a true malt vinegar as they still have some hops in the brewing.

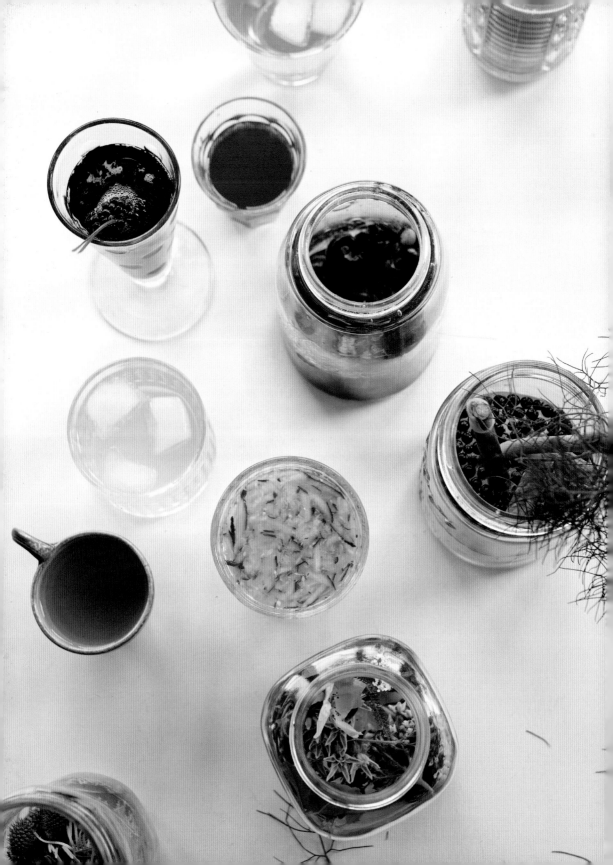

DRINKING VINEGARS

ONCE YOU HAVE A cabinet filled with different vintages and varieties of vinegars, you will want to find ways to enjoy them. And once you understand the variety and complexity of flavors from small-batch fermented vinegars, you'll understand why "drinking vinegars" are a thing. Whether you sip a spritzer, down a switchel after a long, hot day, or enjoy a spirited vinegar cocktail, I hope these recipes open up a world of possibilities for turning your vinegars into delightful beverages. As with anything, though, you don't want to overdo it. Drinking straight vinegar can be hard on your teeth or your stomach.

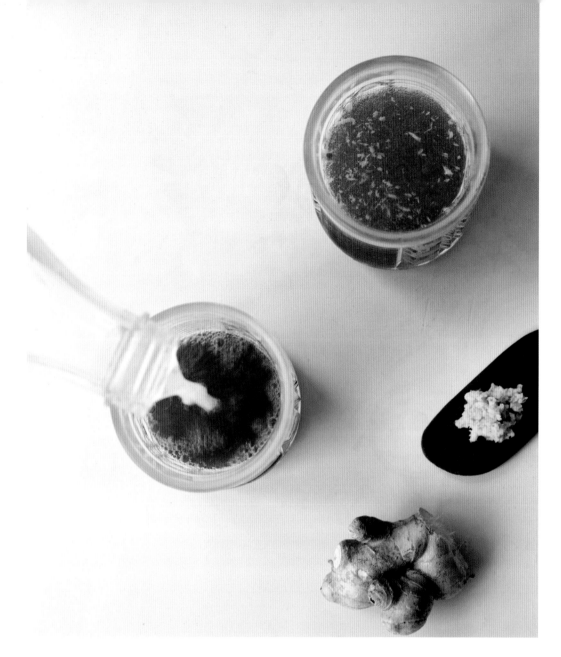

WAYS TO DRINK VINEGAR

Drinking vinegars have a similar history to that of alcohol, in that vinegar was a natural progression in the preservation of fruit. But it was also a strategy for staying hydrated, especially in hot weather, without drinking the water. In the early nineteenth century, it wasn't commonly understood that pathogens in water made people sick. Folks did, however, have an understanding of vinegar's many benefits and its long history as an additive to water; therefore, a popular way to drink water was with vinegar and often other herbs, spices, and sweeteners. Vinegar did help with hydration because there are some electrolytes on board especially when served with sugar, but it also made water tastier, which helped folks drink more. One magazine from this time reads, "when the thermometer ranges among the nineties, it is not so much a question of what we shall eat as what we shall drink."

Spritzers and Spirited Vinegars

Most of our vinegar drinks are nothing fancy: a midmorning pick-me-up spritzer. This simply means putting a splash of straight vinegar into unflavored carbonated water. Many homemade vinegars are mellow and nuanced and can be experienced at their purest this way.

I've developed a riff on drinking vinegars that I'm calling spirited vinegars. These young vinegars are alcoholic beverages in transition and are very drinkable in small amounts, almost like a shot of a distilled liquor. The acid isn't fully developed, and the alcohol is quite diminished. There is nothing wrong with spirits, of course; spirited vinegars are simply another option when we're reaching for a little "something-something" to satisfy a craving. These spirited vinegars can offer some of the pleasures of a harder drink—sensual mouthfeel and a little burn and the happy feeling of a little bevvie—but it stops there. Sorry, no buzz. We enjoy sipping them neat in our favorite highball glasses in the late afternoon or after a rich dinner. Interestingly, feeling happy after a vinegar drink is not as far-fetched as you may think. Vinegar can trigger the breakdown of proteins in the foods you eat into amino acids, which eventually creates tryptophan. Coconut vinegars already have these amino acids on board. The metabolism of tryptophan results in serotonin and melatonin production.

The pleasurable thing about these spirited vinegars is that they are like seasonal foods; they are fleeting in their moment of perfection, and that is part of the magic. Adding anything new to your diet can be uncomfortable. None of my recipe tasters experienced any discomfort with these spirited vinegars; however, please be aware of your own experience. These are also wonderful diluted with bubbly water.

Switchels

When you add sugar, a drinking vinegar is elevated to a switchel or a shrub—the quick distinction between the two is what kind of sugar they contain. Switchel is made with molasses, maple syrup, or some other sweetener, and was sometimes called haymaker's punch, as it was the 1800s version of Gatorade for farmers working long days in the fields.

During the same period, switchel was also a sailor's drink; the hope was that the vinegar and molasses would help hide the taste of the stale, often murky, barreled water. It was thought that if water smelled foul, it was bad. As such, citing "superior efficacy against putrefaction" of the water, Benjamin Morrill Jr., captain of the schooner *Antarctic*, wrote to the Secretary of the US Navy that "ships on long voyages . . . [should] be carefully furnished with a due quantity of vinegar. . . . Switchel, or molasses and water, with a little vinegar in it, should be served out to [sailors] . . . once or twice a day, while at sea." It is thought that ginger was added to the mix to counteract bloating and stomach upsets that could come from drinking too much water. It was believed cold (especially iced) water caused stomach discomfort.

Again, these adjustments were made knowing water could cause issues but without a full understanding why it sometimes did. The acid in the vinegar would lower the pH and take care of many harmful bacteria in the water, but not parasites like giardia. Another benefit was that making the water taste better was good for morale—a huge consideration on the long, hard, days in the cramped quarters of a schooner.

If we look at this water sanitation strategy from the perspective of modern times, we recognize it takes just a modest amount of vinegar to bring the pH below 4.0. But as Reginald Smith (page 19) said, "whether it is officially recognized as making water safe is difficult to say. In practice it probably can in the right amount, but it isn't a standard anyone recognizes."

Switchel was a popular drink during the early years of the United States, but this was by no means a new drink. The ancient Greeks used *oxymel* (which translates as "acid and honey") as medicine, while the Persians were drinking *sharbat-e-sekanjabin* ("honey and vinegar") both as medicine but also as a summer refreshment served with mint. Ancient Roman soldiers (mostly lower ranking) were given *posca* (vinegar diluted with water) for fortitude and strength. It also kept the water safe for days.

Shrubs

Shrubs—such a great word, and not one that refers to the scruffy plants in the sad beds of a parking lot—are sweetened fruit syrups preserved with vinegar. That's it! Recently rediscovered and easy to make, these vinegar syrups are showing up on cocktail menus everywhere. They are quite tasty in adult beverages, but shrubs can be so much more. Add a splash of shrub to a bit of still or bubbly water for a tangy, tart, and sweet, refreshing drink. Or market it to your family as homemade soda.

A basic traditional shrub is made from equal parts fruit, vinegar, and sugar. The chopped or muddled fruit is steeped in vinegar and sugar. I tend to prefer a higher acid ratio for simple nonalcoholic drinks. In fact, I rarely add much sweetener and so am surprised when we buy vinegar drink concentrates and find they are syrupy and very sweet. I also take the fruit flavor up a notch when faced with summer fruit at its peak, such as blackberries, fresh peaches, or strawberries. A modern shrub can also include herbs or spices. The only limit is your imagination.

THE ORIGIN OF SHRUBS

The origin of these vinegar-based syrups goes way back as another way of preserving fruit. As far as we can tell, the history of this drink goes something like this. Most sources agree the word *shrub* comes from *sherbet* (*sharbat-e-sekanjabin*)—not an icy dessert, but the Persian soft drink. It was made from water and vinegar mixed with a sugary fruit mash that had been turned into syrup and dried for convenience while travelling.

In the making of a shrub, the sugar and acidity work in tandem to ensure that the spoiling microbes are kept away for preservation. The fruit can be kept softening and infusing in the vinegar for short periods or for months. Most often, the fruit is strained out at some point, either just before serving or after the infusion is complete.

Our modern shrub hails from England where, in the latter part of the fifteenth century, there emerged a medicinal drink called a cordial. The cordial took on the form of a shrub; the vinegar and fruit–based mixer dealt with the pesky water issues by flavoring and acidifying it. The alcoholic cordial we think of today came about when brandy and rum smugglers in the eighteenth century would hide their casks off the English coast until they could bring them ashore without being seen, in order to avoid taxes. Often these casks would be tainted with a little seawater. To mask the flavor, these spirits were adulterated with sugar and fruit.

This tradition came to the colonies, where shrubs were popular. Benjamin Franklin made a shrub by adding two quarts of orange juice and two pounds of sugar to a gallon of rum. This sat in a casks for a month or so. Martha Washington and notable cookbook authors of the time included a recipe or two for shrub. My copy of an 1897 *White House Cookbook* includes a recipe for raspberry shrub—though it's rum based rather than vinegar based. Use of rum in shrubs would soon diminish, however, as supporters of the temperance movement extolled the virtues of the nonalcoholic shrub as a tasty alternative to alcohol. (I wonder if they realized how tasty shrubs are in cocktails?!)

DRINKING VINEGAR, SHRUB, OR VINEGAR CORDIAL?

The words describing acid-based drinks have become a little blurred. I've noticed that the words *shrub* or *drinking vinegar* and, most recently, *vinegar cordial* on a menu can describe the same concoction. It seems to depend on where you are ordering it. In a bar, the shrub is an ingredient in the cocktail, whereas at a farm-to-table restaurant you might see drinking vinegar on the table. I believe that a vinegar cordial is just a rebranding of the two. My own distinction is that a drinking vinegar is pretty much a delicious unadulterated, or botanically infused, vinegar, in water—but that is just me.

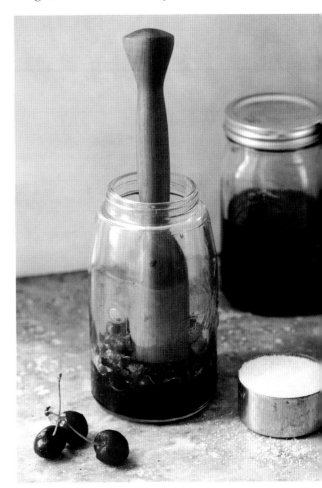

FORAGING FOR FLAVOR:
WILDCRAFTING BOTANICALS

Vinegar is a wonderful medium for capturing and enjoying the flavors and benefits of wild plants. The increasing popularity of foraging, however, has raised a concern about whether wildcrafting is sustainable. Here are a few tips for how to harvest responsibly.

HARVEST WILD EDIBLES SPARINGLY. Fortunately, when you're foraging for plants to infuse in vinegars, you don't need to harvest a huge quantity. Take less than half of any given plant or even less if there is only a small population. If you are harvesting wild yeast (page 53) you can pick a blossom or two. One small cluster of milkweed flowers, for example, will give you enough yeast and essence for a couple of quarts of vinegar.

GIVE BACK TO THE LANDSCAPE. Learn how to propagate the wild plants you love, and if you have space, plant your favorites in your home garden. Or simply collect seeds in fall and plant them in the wild.

COLLECT INVASIVE AND DOMESTICATED PLANTS. Feel free to use as many invasive plants as you like! And don't forget that domesticated plants—for example, the petals of sunflowers or roses in the garden, or any garden herbs—have flavor to offer, too.

AVOID HARVESTING PLANTS GROWING BY ROADSIDES. These may contain harmful chemicals. Similarly, don't harvest from plants that have been sprayed with pesticides. Spend some time observing the areas you are interested in harvesting from, and make sure the plants aren't contaminated.

DO YOUR RESEARCH. Know which plants are rare and shouldn't be harvested at all, and don't harvest from protected areas. Identify plants

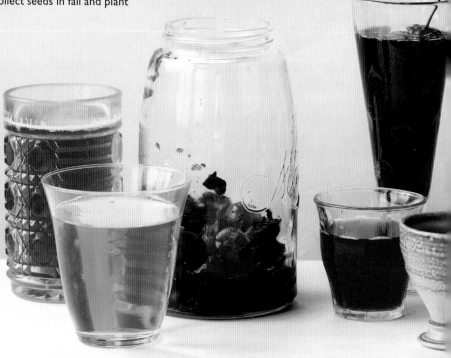

carefully, and harvest only those that are edible or have edible parts.

CONSUME WILDCRAFTED PLANTS SPARINGLY. Use just a small quantity of flowers and botanicals—at first, especially—as some may cause digestive upset in some people.

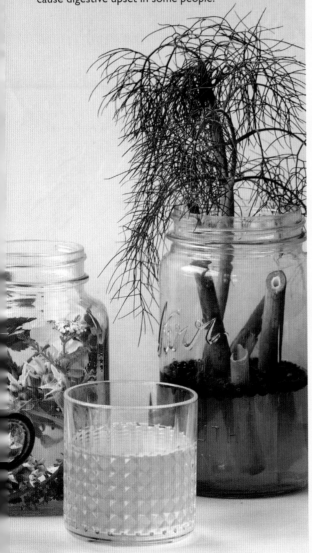

HOW MUCH VINEGAR CAN I DRINK?

Chapter 10 covers some of the purported benefits of drinking vinegar as tonics or teas— simply a few teaspoons of vinegar diluted with water and honey, ginger, or other ingredients. The health benefits of drinking vinegar, how- ever, are not backed up by a lot of research. Christopher and I view the vinegars I make as another food: a delicious expression of fer- mentation and healthy, whole ingredients. As such, these manifestations of plant and time make delicious beverages.

The answer to the question "How much can I drink?" is "It depends." As with anything, one person's cure is another person's poison. We need to pay attention to what our bodies tell us. Christopher and I have never experienced problems from drinking vinegar. However, all of us are different. For example, if you have acid reflux or a compromised digestive system, vinegar could aggravate it—or cure it. Acid reflux has many different causes depending on the person. If the cause is low stomach acid (hypochlorhydria), then a bit of vinegar in water before a meal can be an amazing simple cure. This is because it both introduces acid into the digestive tract as well as acts as an antimicrobial. (Interestingly, low stomach acid allows the wrong bacteria to have a large pop- ulation. These bacteria feed on carbs, causing the bubbling and discomfort in your stomach.) However, for others, as our friend and craft vinegar maker Jitti Chaithiraphant said, it's "like throwing gasoline on a fire." You should also be aware that drinking undiluted vinegar can harm the enamel on your teeth.

We cannot tell you how much the right amount for you is, or how much is too much. We do advocate balance and moderation in everything and, especially, trusting your gut.

Base Recipe for a Modern Drinking Vinegar

THIS RECIPE IS FOR making a drinking vinegar that is not based on fruit, as the shrub is. Instead it's based on the flavor of the vinegar itself, adorned with herbs and other botanicals. This is truly your adventure; what flavors do you like? Maybe try making seasonal vinegars, using spicy flavors in the winter and light, bright flavors in the summer. I like wildcrafting with the seasons; it's a way I can feel more in tune with the cycles of the year.

YIELD
about 1 quart

Handful of botanicals (herbs, flowers, spices, fir tips)

1 quart (0.9 L) vinegar

Unrefined demerara sugar, honey, or maple syrup (optional)

1. Put the botanicals into a sanitized jar. Pour the vinegar over the top.

2. Place the lid on the jar, tighten, and let the jar sit on the counter for 2 to 4 weeks.

3. When the vinegar is ready, strain the solids through a piece of cheesecloth placed in a sieve or colander. Squeeze out all the vinegar.

4. Add the sugar or other sweetener, and stir until dissolved.

5. Transfer the finished vinegar to a jar or pretty bottle that has an airtight seal. Sealed tightly, it will last several months to a year or more in a cool, dark cabinet.

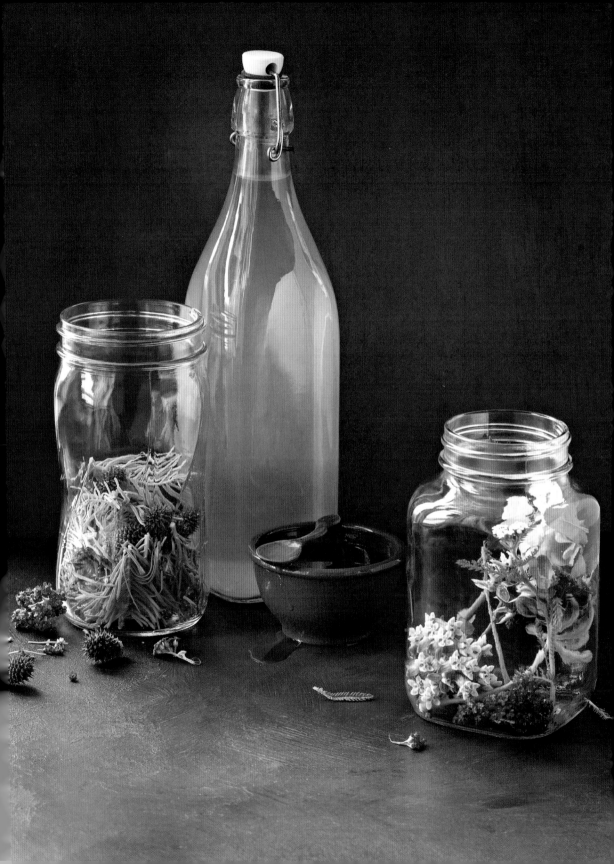

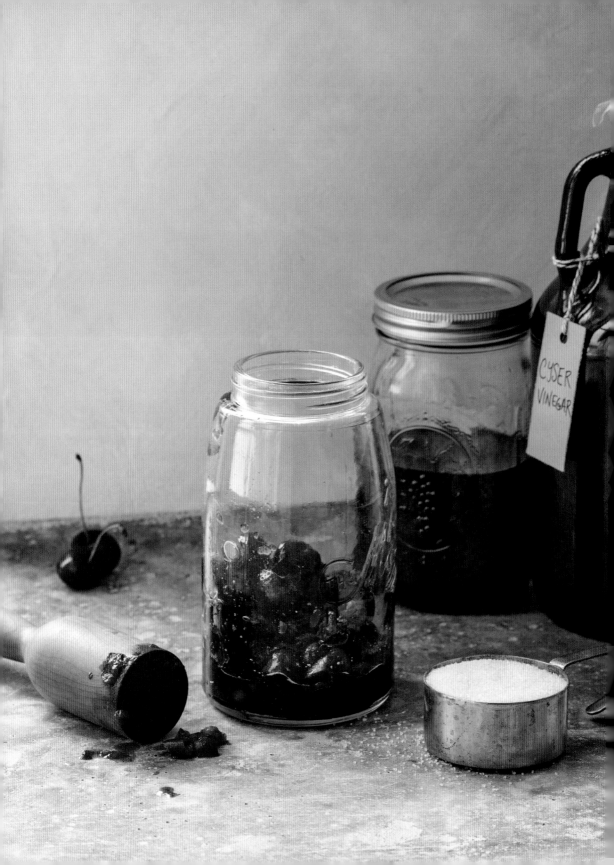

Base Recipe for a Modern Shrub

USE YOUR HOMEMADE VINEGAR to preserve whatever shrub-making ingredients you have on hand, from berries to ripe tomatoes. If you leave the shrub out at room temperature, it will oxidize more, changing the flavors. In the refrigerator it will last up to a year.

YIELD
about 1 quart

2⅔ cups (415 g) fresh fruit (the juicier the better), seeded or pitted

1 cup (200 g) sugar or another sweetener

2 cups (473 mL) cider vinegar

Sparkling mineral water, seltzer, club soda, or water, to serve

1. Slice, chop, or pulse the fruit quickly in food processor. Place the fruit and sugar in a sanitized half-gallon jar. Use a wooden spoon (or muddler) to crush the fruit. Allow it to sit in the refrigerator for 24 hours to macerate, stirring occasionally.

2. Strain the fruit from the juice through a fine-meshed sieve, or cheesecloth draped in a colander, over a large bowl. Give the liquid time to drip out. If you want your shrub clear, don't press or squeeze the fruit. If you want a cloudy shrub and a little fiber (always a good thing), squeeze the cheesecloth enough so that you get some fine fruit pulp in the liquid. To that end, if you want all the fiber, don't strain at all, just run the whole thing through a blender until puréed. Full utilization tip: Add the leftover fruit to fresh apples or other fruit for a crisp or cobbler.

3. Combine the fruit syrup with the vinegar in a jar or pretty bottle that has an air-tight seal. Store in the refrigerator, where it will last for several months to a year.

4. To serve as a nonalcoholic bubbly drink, add one part of your shrub to three or four parts bubbly water—sparkling mineral water, seltzer, club soda, or the stuff you make in your soda machine. You can, of course, use still water. But let's be real: Most of us like bubbles.

Boiled Cider
(a.k.a. Cider Syrup)

BOILED CIDER IS SIMPLY apple cider that has been reduced to apple syrup. It is a delicious sweetener for shrubs and other vinegar drinks. Anyone who has tasted fresh-boiled cider may argue that it is more than just syrup. It has complex sweet-sour flavors; it is tart apple pie and maple syrup. It is pure apple sugar bliss. Any apple juice will work, but ideally use freshly pressed apple juice because it is thicker and richer. If you press your own, try a mix of apple varieties with different levels of acidity to balance out the sugar, to make a syrup that is more appley than just flatly sweet. This same reduction technique can be used with any kind of fruit juice. I often make a sour cherry syrup in the same manner.

YIELD
2–2½ cups

1   gallon (3.8 L) or more apple juice

1.   Pour the juice into a nonreactive pot and slowly bring to a simmer over low heat. The wider the pot the better, as this gives the cider more surface area to evaporate, allowing the whole process to take less time.

2.   Lower the heat to keep the cider at a constant simmer. If you keep it below 140°F/60°C, it will not candy. When the cider simmers, you will notice that it separates—the clear liquid from some brown solids. At this point, you can remove the solids with a skimmer or strain the cider through a piece of muslin for a clear syrup. Up to you.

3.   Stir the cider now and then, more often as it thickens and nears the last 45 minutes of the cooking time, to keep it from scorching. You will know it is ready when it is the consistency of maple syrup and coats the spoon. Cooking time, in general, is 4 to 5 hours.

4.   Ladle the syrup into hot, sterilized jars, leaving ¼-inch headspace, and can them in a hot-water bath for 5 minutes. Alternatively, seal tightly and store in the refrigerator indefinitely.

Spiced Apple Shrub

THIS IS A WARM and toasty winter-evening shrub. It will make a refreshing bubbly spritzer or a variation on hot buttered rum. We heat the vinegar, as it brings out more flavor in the spices. However, if you prefer to keep it raw, simply start with step 2.

YIELD
1 quart

1¾ cups (414 mL) cider vinegar

1 3- to 4-inch (8 to 10 cm) cinnamon stick

1 teaspoon (2 g) ground ginger

¼ teaspoon (1 g) grated nutmeg

1–2 whole cloves

2¼ cups (532 mL) boiled cider (page 238)

Sparkling mineral water, seltzer, club soda, or water, to serve

1. Combine the vinegar, cinnamon, ginger, nutmeg, and cloves in a small nonreactive saucepan. Bring to a simmer over medium heat. Turn off the heat and let sit until cool.

2. Pour the spiced-vinegar mixture into a clean jar, attach a tight-fitting lid, and let marinate for 3 days.

3. Strain out the spices with a fine-mesh sieve, or cheesecloth draped in a colander, over a bowl.

4. Combine the clear spiced vinegar with the boiled cider in a sanitized jar or pretty bottle that has an airtight seal. Store in the refrigerator, where it will last for several months to a year.

5. To serve as a nonalcoholic bubbly drink, add one part of your shrub to three or four parts sparkling or still water.

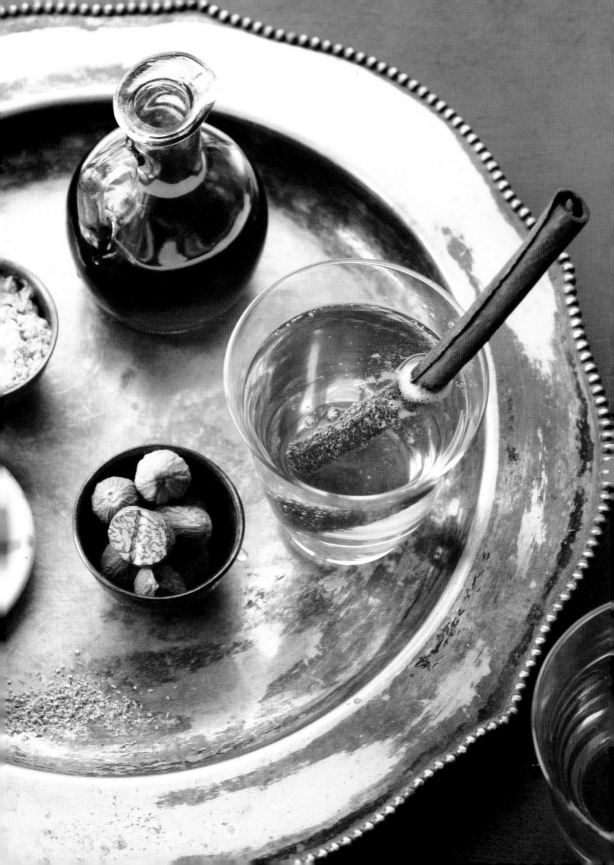

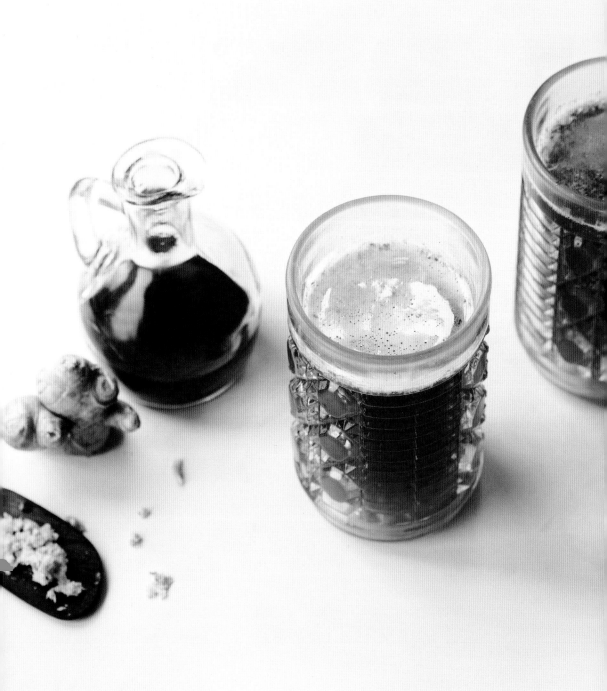

Classic Switchel

THIS IS MORE FORMULA than recipe. Use it as a jumping-off point to exercise your creativity, and feel free to drop in other spices, herbs, or fruit. Traditionally, this is made with apple cider vinegar. When I'm sweetening with molasses, I do prefer the flavor and acid of ACV. Other fruit vinegars lend themselves to lighter sweeteners, like maple syrup (try it with white wine vinegar or pear vinegar). See page 215 for a hot molasses tea that came directly from the idea of a switchel drink.

YIELD
about 1 quart

2   cups (473 mL) apple cider vinegar or other vinegar of your choice

2   cups (473 mL) maple syrup, or molasses, or honey, or 2 cups (400 g) brown or other unrefined cane sugar

1   ounce (28 g) freshly grated ginger, or 1 teaspoon (12 g) dry ground ginger

Still or sparkling water, to serve

1. Stir together the vinegar, sweetener, and ginger in a quart jar with lid. Mix well. Tighten lid. Use immediately or store in a cabinet for several months, or in the refrigerator for a year or more.

2. To serve, add just a few tablespoons per cup of still or sparkling, warm or cold water, or use any ratio you like.

FEEL THE BURN

Interestingly eighteenth-century thinkers surmised that hot drinks were healthier refreshments while working in the sun, to maintain the body's balance. Hydration was not yet a concept. Beverages with both ginger's spicy bite and alcohol's burn fell into the category of "hot" drinks to maintain equilibrium. When the temperance movement came around in the nineteenth century, the ginger switchel was rebranded as a replacement for the burn of alcohol.

Honey Sekanjabin

THIS REFRESHING DRINK is an ancient Persian forerunner to a shrub or switchel called *sharbat-e-sekanjabin*. Like an oxymel (page 270), it was used medicinally. Ancient Persian texts describe more than 1,200 vinegar and honey combinations complete with considerations and contraindications. This drink is still popular in Iran today, where it is served with shredded cucumber and tender lettuce leaves. Although the modern Iranian preparation uses white sugar syrup, to which the vinegar and mint are added, the ancient sweetener was honey.

Every recipe I found required boiling the sugar or honey syrup, but there is some evidence that heating honey damages its antimicrobial properties and can cause it to become carcinogenic. This variation is a cool process and takes a little longer to make, but the resultant syrup stores for months in the refrigerator.

YIELD
about 1½ cups

1 cup (237 mL) vinegar of your choice

1 bunch (about 90 g) fresh mint, or about 3 tablespoons (3 g) dried

2 cups (680 g) honey

Grated cucumber, for serving

1. Pour the vinegar into a nonreactive saucepan and heat over low heat to warm slightly, to about 135°F/57°C. Watch it carefully: You don't want to cook it at all. This is just to help get those enzymes to break down the herbs.

2. Finely chop the mint, stems and all, and put in a sanitized pint jar.

3. Pour your warmed vinegar over the herbs. They should be completely covered. Stir them in to make sure they are all submerged.

4. Screw on the jar lid, slipping a bit of parchment paper between the jar and the metal lid to prevent corrosion.

5. Place the jar on your counter (but out of direct sunlight) so you remember to shake it every few days to redistribute the contents. Let it infuse for 2 weeks.

6. After 2 weeks, strain out the herbs. Line a strainer with a piece of butter muslin or fine-mesh cheesecloth and strain the mixture into a new sanitized jar. Squeeze the cloth to get every last tasty drop out. (Set the pickled herbs aside to refrigerate in a small jar for another use—salad dressing, garnish, you get the idea.)

7. Pour the honey into a bowl, add the infused vinegar, and mix well. When thoroughly mixed, transfer the honey vinegar to a storage jar with a noncorrosive lid. This mixture will last indefinitely if refrigerated.

8. To prepare the sekanjabin, mix about six parts water to one part syrup. Pour over ice and add about ¼ cup grated cucumber to each glass.

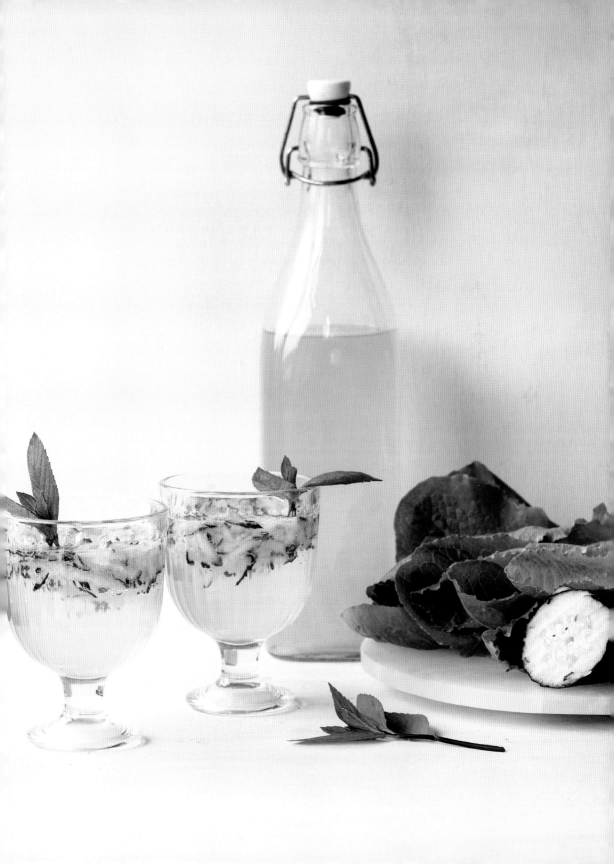

Base Recipe for Spirited Vinegar

YOU'VE MET A VARIATION of this recipe for the kitchen-counter Boerhaave method for speeding up vinegar fermentation. Here I present it again as a way to brew drinking vinegar. Use your imagination! Remember that as long as the filler material isn't toxic, it's fair game—what about pine sticks for a vinegar riff on retsina? Or dried citrus peels (with a sweet cider) for a limoncello? Let your imagination go wild.

YIELD
about 2 quarts

Filler material as needed to fill a 1-quart jar about ⅔ full

½–1 cup (118–237 mL) raw, unfiltered, unpasteurized vinegar

1 quart plus 1 cup (1.2 L) hard cider

1. Evenly divide the filler material between two sanitized 1-quart jars, so that each is one-third full. Pour the vinegar over the filler in one jar until it is covered, and let marinate for an hour or two. Pour off the vinegar into the second jar and repeat the soaking time. Drain the remaining vinegar (whatever has not been soaked up by the filler) from the second jar, strain it, and bottle to store or use. Alternatively, you can put the vinegar in one of the jars and it will become part of the new vinegar.

2. Fill one jar to the top with the cider. This will give you the starting amount. Now pour out about one-quarter of that cider into the second jar. This will leave you with one jar that is three-quarters full and another that is one-quarter full.

3. Cover the jar with a piece of unbleached cotton (butter muslin or tightly woven cheesecloth), or a basket-style paper coffee filter. Secure with a string, a rubber band, or a threaded metal canning band. This is to keep out fruit flies.

4. Place the jars in a spot that is warm (ideally 75° to 86°F/25° to 30°C; see page 71 for more specifics on temperature) and convenient, because you will be working with them daily.

5. The next day, pour the liquid from the nearly full jar into the other jar, leaving about one-fourth in the bottom of the first jar, exposing most of the filler material. This will move oxygen through the liquid and give the bacteria on the filler material time to "breathe." Do this once daily or two to three times a day to speed the process. Over the next few days, the filler will continue to absorb liquid and swell. As this happens, add more cider, if needed, to keep one jar full and the other at that quarter mark.

6. In a few days, you will start to smell the distinctive vinegar aroma. Continue to transfer the mixture from jar to jar. Assuming a once-daily transfer at room temperature, in about 7 days you will have a mighty fine spirited, half-finished vinegar. Take some off the top and enjoy it, replacing what you withdrew with more cider. You can keep this up indefinitely for a continuous daily "cocktail."

7. Alternatively, you can bottle it as is. To hold the flavor longer, pasteurize the liquid or keep it in the refrigerator, sealed. This spirited vinegar is alive. The microbes are still hard at work, so it's a race to hold back the oxygen and consume the beverage before they do.

8. To create finished vinegar, keep the process going instead of immediately bottling. In 3 to 5 weeks, you should have a finished vinegar. After the first round, the process will be faster because the filler material will be fully inoculated. In fact, at some point you will see bits of a mother forming on the filler. Traditionally, this is removed because it gets in the way. But if you will be making many batches from the same filler, pick off the mother—or leave it if you think it's cool. It won't cause harm.

9. Bottle the finished vinegar. Use immediately, or age to allow it to mellow and develop flavors.

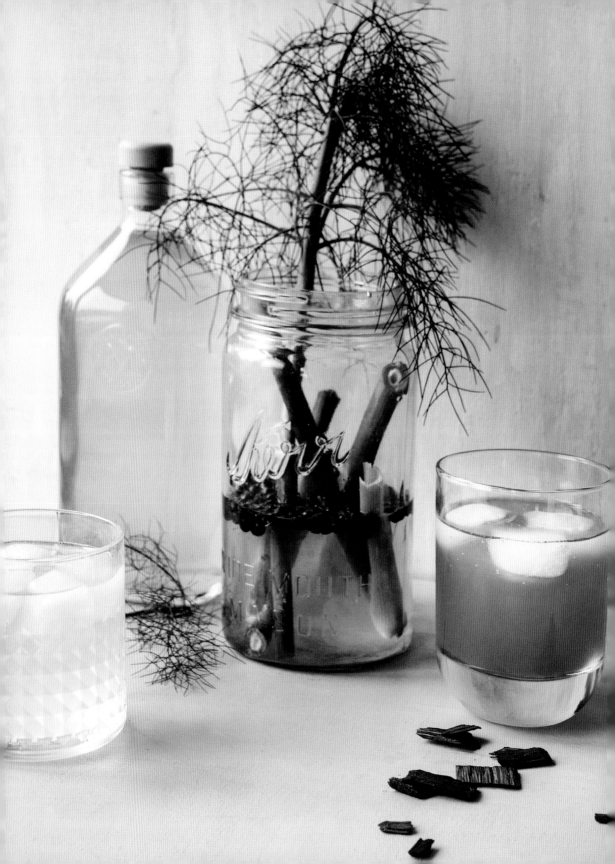

Bourbon-Style "Drink"-ing Vinegar

THIS IS ANOTHER Boerhaave-method drinking vinegar. I like using oak chips (charred or not) for the filler material because of the barrel-aged flavor it imparts. Feel free to experiment with different woods, as they'll each impart their own qualities. You can also find oak cubes or spirals that have been charred for brewing at brewing suppliers.

Charring wood creates tannins, terpenes, and volatile compounds; this creates unique flavors, like the vanilla flavor in bourbon. It might sound crazy, but after a week of being on the oak, a half-finished vinegar gives the mouth an experience similar to that of sipping a nice whiskey: that burn on the back of the throat and the long, lingering taste of vanilla oak filling your mouth when the burn has settled.

YIELD
about ½ gallon

- 3 cups oak chips, or more as needed
- 2–4 cups (473–946 mL) raw , unfiltered, unpasteurized vinegar
- 3 quarts (2.8 L) hard cider

1. Evenly divide the chips between two sanitized half-gallon jars so that each is one-third full. Pour the vinegar over the chips of one jar until they are covered. Let the chips marinate for an hour or two. Pour off the vinegar into the second jar. Repeat the soaking time. Strain any vinegar that is left, and bottle to store or use. Alternatively, you can put the vinegar in one of the two jars and it will become part of the new vinegar.

2. Fill one jar to the top with the cider. This will give you the starting amount. Now pour out about one-quarter of cider into the second jar. This will leave you with one jar that is three-quarters full and another that is one-quarter full.

3. Cover the jars with pieces of unbleached cotton (butter muslin or tightly woven cheesecloth), or basket-style paper coffee filters. Secure with strings, rubber bands, or threaded metal canning bands. This is to keep out fruit flies.

4. Place the jars in a spot that is warm (ideally 75° to 86°F/25° to 30°C; see page 71) and convenient, because you will be working with them daily.

recipe continues on next page

5. The next day, pour the liquid from the nearly full jar into the other jar, leaving about one-fourth in the bottom of the first jar, exposing most of the filler material. This will move oxygen through the liquid and give the bacteria on the filler material time to "breathe." Do this once daily or two to three times a day to speed the process. Over the next few days, the chips will continue to absorb liquid and swell. As this happens, add more cider, if needed, to keep one jar full and the other at that quarter mark.

6. In a few days, you will start to smell the distinctive vinegar aroma. Continue to transfer the mixture from jar to jar. Assuming a once-daily transfer at room temperature, in about 7 days you will have a mighty fine spirited, half-finished vinegar. Take some off the top and enjoy it, replacing what you withdrew with more cider. You can keep this up indefinitely for a continuous daily "cocktail."

7. Alternatively, you can bottle it as is. To hold the flavor longer, pasteurize the liquid or keep it in the refrigerator sealed. This spirited vinegar is alive. The microbes are still hard at work, so it's a race to hold back the oxygen and consume the beverage before they do.

8. To create finished vinegar, keep the process going instead of immediately bottling. In 3 to 5 weeks, you should have a finished vinegar. After the first round, the process will be faster because the chips are now fully inoculated. In fact, at some point you will see bits of a mother forming on the chips. Traditionally, this is removed because it gets in the way. But if you will be making many batches from the same filler chips, pick off the mother or leave it if you think it's cool. It won't cause harm.

9. Bottle the finished vinegar. Use immediately, or age to allow it to mellow and flavors to develop.

Variation:
Gin Botanical
Spirited Vinegar

IF GIN IS MORE YOUR PREFERENCE than whiskey, try adding gin botanicals. Juniper is the main botanical used in gin, and so fennel stalks replace the oak chips in this recipe, to add a complementary flavor. Follow the process above, using two 1-quart jars. The biggest difference is that we soak the fennel stalks and juniper but remove all the starter vinegar, because we want the finished vinegar to be as clear as possible.

3 tablespoons (11 g) juniper berries, crushed lightly

6–8 fennel stalks, dried

5 cups (1.2 L) clear light semisweet hard cider or white wine
(plus 1 cup/237 mL water if using wine)

1 cup (237 mL) raw white wine vinegar or apple cider vinegar

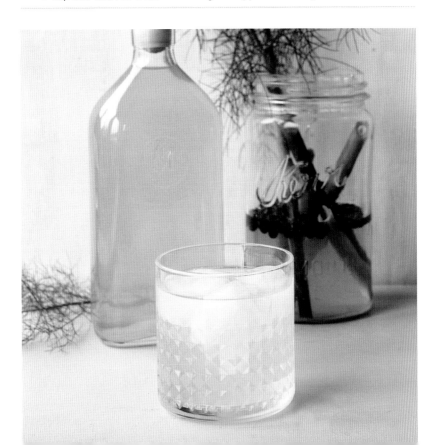

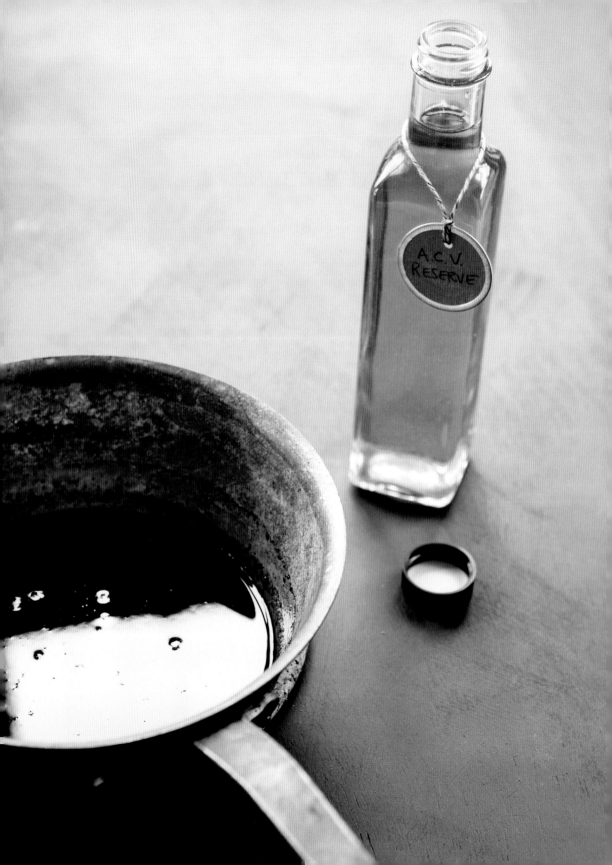

Cider Shrub

THIS RECIPE IS APPLE SQUARED. It came about when I was trying to come up with a shortcut to a thick, balsamic-type apple vinegar. I made an extra-thick boiled cider, with the intention that it would thicken and sweeten vinegar for an approximation of classic, rich balsamic. This didn't result in anything that resembled a hack to an apple balsamic, but it did become a delicious drinking vinegar.

YIELD
about 1 quart

2¼ cups (534 mL) boiled cider (page 238)

1¾ cups (414 mL) cider vinegar

   Sparkling mineral water, club soda, or water, to serve

1. Combine the boiled cider and vinegar in a sanitized jar or pretty bottle. Store in the refrigerator. It will last for several months to a year.

2. Time to enjoy. If you want a nonalcoholic bubbly drink, add one part of your shrub to three or four parts still or sparkling water.

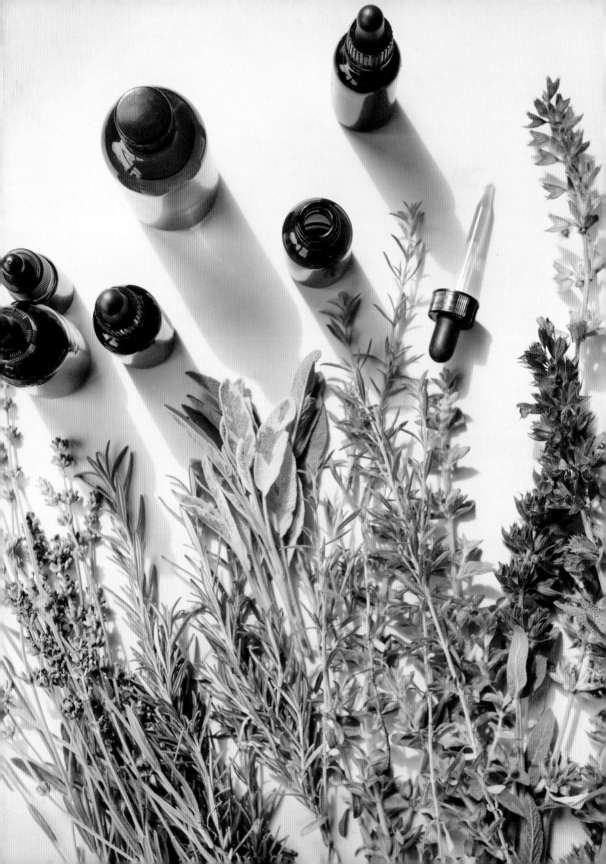

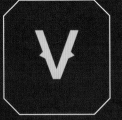

VINEGAR IS AN original member of the "food is medicine" club and has long been used in traditional medicine to treat a wide variety of ailments. It's commonly touted now as an appetite suppressant to assist with weight loss. Its acidity helps our digestive systems do a better job of absorbing minerals and balancing the body's pH. It can improve insulin sensitivity in diabetics, keeping blood sugar levels in check by keeping the body from fully digesting starch. Other popular applications include controlling bad breath or candida, cancer prevention, protecting from heart disease, and more. Add to that external uses including hair and skin products, and an online search on the health benefits of vinegar might feel like watching a tennis match as the theories are lobbed back and forth between cure-all and snake oil. As always, the answer lies somewhere in between. All that aside, there is enough evidence to include raw vinegar as part of a healthy diet, combined with observing your own body's reaction to using any food as medicine to guide you.

VINEGAR AND TRADITIONAL KNOWLEDGE

People around the world have used vinegar for medicine throughout history. There isn't an ancient culture—from China to India, Persia, and westward to Egypt, Greece, and Rome—that doesn't mention vinegar's healing properties in its materia medica. For example, the five-volume *Al-Qanun fi al-Tibb* (*The Canon of Medicine*) by Persian physician Ibn Sina, completed in 1025, contains numerous treatments.

Historically, vinegar has been used as a "functional food"—something that is considered both food and medicine—just as honey, hot peppers, turmeric, ginger, and many other foods have been. But despite vinegar's long history as both a food and a medicine, with a large body of literature to support this, modern scientific research has not fully examined its medicinal qualities. Guided by just a handful of studies—as well as thousands of years of traditional knowledge—our use of vinegar is very much part of a rich, whole-food diet that includes cooking whole foods and eating traditionally fermented preparations.

Antibacterial Qualities

Vinegar has long been valued for its antibacterial qualities. The tenth-century creator of forensic medicine, Sung Tse, advocated hand washing with sulfur and vinegar to avoid infection during autopsies. Hippocrates recommended vinegar for treating sores and cleaning wounds. Vinegar played an important role during the plague (see page 262). Twelfth-century nun and physician Hildegard von Bingen wrote, "Vinegar purifies the stinking in

man and makes sure that his food is in the right path."

This antibacterial property comes mostly from vinegar's acidity. Autopsies and plagues aside, this is how humans have been able to safely preserve foodstuffs for lean times. On fresh greens, this acidity can have immediate benefits. A study in 2005 evaluated vinegar's antimicrobial qualities by inoculating arugula greens and sliced spring onions with salmonella, then putting vinegar, lemon juice, or a combination of the two, on these salmonella salads. Both the vinegar and lemon juice significantly decreased the concentrations of salmonella, and the combination of the two acids made the salmonella undetectable.[10] Go acid!

This strong action against the bad bacteria doesn't affect the good bacteria, fortunately, because the good guys don't mind the acidity. In fact, vinegar may even enhance levels of good bacteria. For example, researchers found mice that were fed vinegar in their water had higher levels of good bacteria, such as lactobacillus and bifidobacteria, in their guts.

Digestive and Cardiovascular Effects

Historically, "vinegar teas" (which are basically warm vinegar drinks, with or without herbs) were a common way for diabetics to manage their condition.[11] There is some evidence that it lowers blood sugar, and for folks with type 2 diabetes or insulin resistance, a dose of vinegar before a meal improves the insulin sensitivity and responses to a high carb meal.[12] This premeal dose in water can also stimulate digestion. The extra acid can help the digestive system absorb more nutrients from food. There are a few studies that suggest appetite suppression. There are also a few studies, mostly on animals, that point to lowering blood pressure and reducing the risk of heart disease. Coincidentally, this is consistent with the sixteenth-century Chinese medical writings of Li Shizhen, who recommended vinegar for improving circulation.

Other Health Benefits

Vinegar contains high levels of polyphenols, which are important antioxidants. There are also amino acids in many vinegars, which are known to help reduce muscle cramping and fatigue. It is believed that these daily doses of vinegar and water help keep the circulation in good working order, hold arthritis at bay, and flush toxins from the body.

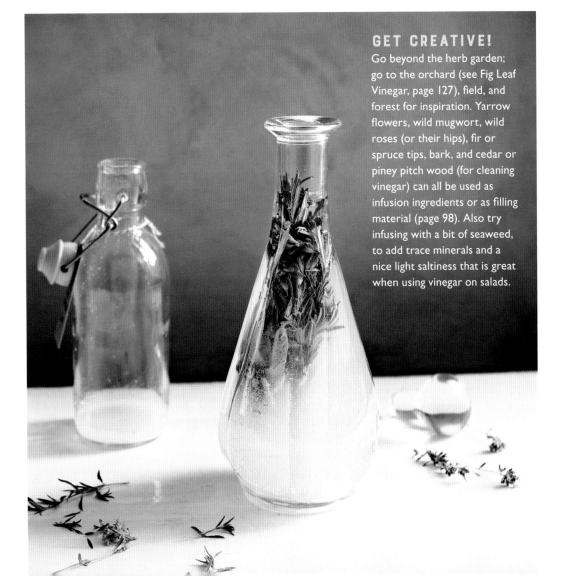

GET CREATIVE!
Go beyond the herb garden; go to the orchard (see Fig Leaf Vinegar, page 127), field, and forest for inspiration. Yarrow flowers, wild mugwort, wild roses (or their hips), fir or spruce tips, bark, and cedar or piney pitch wood (for cleaning vinegar) can all be used as infusion ingredients or as filling material (page 98). Also try infusing with a bit of seaweed, to add trace minerals and a nice light saltiness that is great when using vinegar on salads.

How much vinegar is safe to consume? I was able to find little evidence of risk of regular ingestion, but it should be taken diluted in meals or in water. Most important, when adding vinegar to your diet as a tonic, you should always pay attention to changes in how you feel—good or bad. This will inform your decision about whether you want to continue to consume vinegar.

VINEGAR INFUSIONS

Herb-infused vinegars offer both culinary and medicinal benefits. Often the line between the two can be blurred, as all herbs, whether we classify them as "culinary" or "medicinal," often land in both camps. The beauty of this is that you can have your medicine and eat it, too!

In this chapter, you will find techniques and ideas for infusing herbal vinegars for flavor, medicine, and home uses. After the infusion, you can choose to leave the herbs in the jar or strain them out. In general, these vinegars are at their best if used within six months. While vinegar infusions last indefinitely, some of the infused flavors will fade, which makes sense if you read the section on aging vinegar and how the flavors mellow.

Fermenting Herbs While Making Vinegar

You can ferment any herb while making your vinegar. If you are already making vinegar, it is fun to play around with making herbal vinegars as part of the process. The flavor components come out in a different way altogether. I don't advocate one over the other, but I do encourage playing around with both techniques, with whatever ingredients you have on hand. I often do this as part of the kitchen-counter Boerhaave method on page 94, where the herbal stalks or botanical material become the filler material.

Fresh or Dried?

Some herbalists say only fresh herbs will do, while others say dry is fine. Ultimately, you should use what you have or what is available to you. When choosing fresh herbs or botanicals, make sure they are clean and dry, without damaged or dark spots.

The truth is that not everyone has access to fresh herbs. Don't let this stop you from making an herbal vinegar. When choosing dried herbs, be sure they are from a recent crop. You don't want to use dried herbs that have already lost their punch. Choose a reputable company to order from, as this will ensure a better quality and high enough turnover to have fresher stock. After infusing with dried herbs, you strain the vinegar through a coffee filter or a few layers of cheesecloth. Alternatively, you can place dried herbs in a cloth infusion bag before adding them to the vinegar.

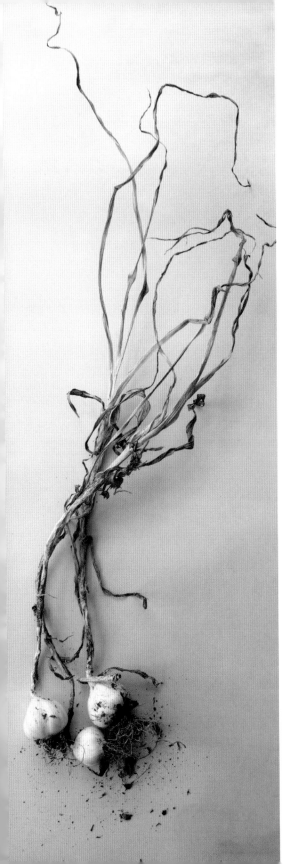

Vinegar Reduction Infusion

A vinegar reduction is a bold herbal vinegar infusion that is more about using vinegar to extract and preserve the herbs (like you would with a tincture) than about kitchen flavor. This method is best used for roots and other hearty herbs. I also use this for whole spices like cloves, allspice, cinnamon sticks, and the like, when I want a flavoring vinegar for mustard. The process is a little harsh for delicate floral and aromatic herbs, as the aromatics will dissipate in the heat. A good rule is to use one part herb to four parts vinegar. This infusion can be used to make an oxymel (page 270). To do so, add equal parts raw honey and infused vinegar.

1. Combine the herbs in a large pot with double the amount of vinegar you intend to end up with. Heat to a gentle simmer. Through reduction, you will lose half the water to evaporation. Warning: The steam coming off the simmering reduction is strong and can be uncomfortable if you put your face over it, especially to your eyes, and to your lungs, if you breathe it in.

2. The infusion will be ready when the volume is about half of the original, which will take 30 to 40 minutes. When finished, let cool, then strain out herbs. Store in an airtight bottle or jar, with a glass and rubber-seal bail-type top or a plastic lid that will not corrode over time. If you don't have either, place parchment paper, waxed cloth, or plastic wrap between the vinegar and the lid.

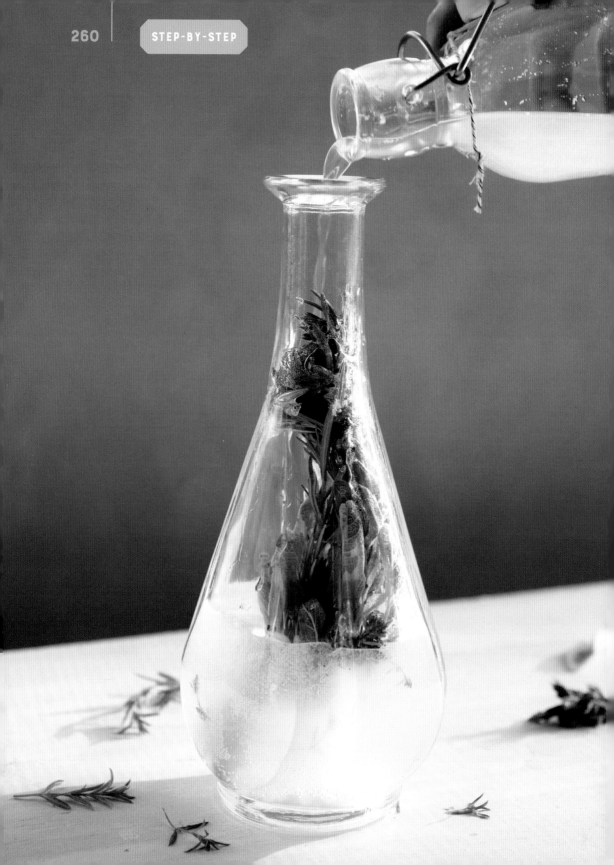

Basic Culinary Vinegar Infusion

Besides cooking with this infusion, you can use it with honey and warm or bubbly water as an instant oxymel (page 270). To do so, add equal parts raw honey and infused vinegar, or to taste.

1. Chop any of the fresh herbs or vegetables into small pieces; use spices whole. Place all the ingredients in a sanitized jar. (Use a glass-topped, rubber-seal, bail-type jar if you have one, to avoid corrosion of the lid.) The herbs should fill about one-third of the jar. If you are using bulkier vegetables, fill to about half of the jar.

2. Warm apple cider vinegar or other homemade vinegar by pouring the amount you will need (3 to 3½ cups [710 to 828 mL]) for a quart jar (0.9 L) in a nonreactive pot on low heat. Alternatively, you can place the bottle in an oven or bread-proofing box set to low. The goal is to the warm it to about 120°F/49°C so that the vinegar will do a good job pulling out the benefits from your herbs.

3. Pour the warmed vinegar over the herbs to fill the jar.

4. Tighten a plastic lid, or a regular lid with a piece of parchment paper, waxed cloth, or plastic wrap between the metal and the mixture to avoid corrosion. Shake the mixture.

5. Place the jar on the counter but out of direct sunlight. Shake every few days to redistribute the herbs. Allow to infuse for at least 2 weeks.

6. Once infused, strain out the herbs or botanicals through a coffee filter or a few layers of cheesecloth and bottle the liquid. Toss the soaked herbs into the compost or, better yet, save to flavor a chutney or other condiment. Store the infusion in a cool, dark place.

Rosemary Gladstar's Four Thieves Vinegar

FOUR THIEVES VINEGAR is a legendary formula, believed to have originated in the fourteenth century, during a devastating bubonic plague pandemic. According to the legend, there were four young grave robbers who were able to avoid the plague (despite their occupation) by taking their mother's herbal remedy. They were eventually caught and, upon threat of hanging, shared the formula. It has changed a bit over the centuries, but the core formulation remains essentially the same. Here's Rosemary Gladstar's (see page 266) favorite version of the recipe, which she has graciously allowed me to share with you. All herbs listed are best used fresh. Chopping the herbs increases the surface area exposed to the vinegar.

6–12 garlic cloves, finely chopped

½ cup (20 g) fresh lavender

½ cup (20 g) fresh rosemary

½ cup (20 g) fresh sage

¼ cup (10 g) fresh thyme

1–2 teaspoons (2.2–4.4 g) ground cloves (see Note)

Apple cider vinegar (raw, unfiltered, and unpasteurized)

1. Combine the garlic, lavender, rosemary, sage, thyme, and cloves in a sanitized widemouthed glass jar. Fill the jar with enough vinegar to cover the herbs by 2 to 3 inches. Cover tightly and let sit in a warm spot for 3 to 4 weeks.

2. Strain out the herbs. Rebottle the vinegar. Store in a cool, dark location, where it will keep for at least a year and usually much longer.

3. Use the vinegar liberally as a flavoring agent in dressings, marinades, and other recipes. Or follow Rosemary's advice and take 1 to 2 tablespoons every 3 to 4 hours to ward off illness.

NOTE: Cloves add a strong flavor not liked by everyone, but according to Rosemary, they contain powerful antimicrobial properties. If you're not a fan of clove, start with a smaller amount and go easy on it.

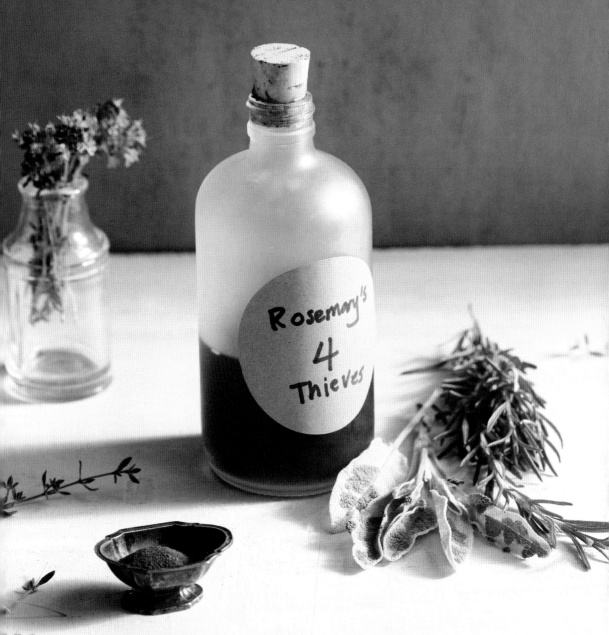

MAKING BOTANICAL VINEGARS FOR GIFTS

- Start saving attractive and interesting bottles. (See Worthy Bottles, page 108.)

- Use plastic or wax-sealed corks for caps, as metal will corrode. Rubber-ringed bail-top jars work well also.

- Bottle the finished vinegar without the original infused botanicals. Leave the vinegar clear or add one new sprig of the herb or botanical. This way, the plant material will be fresh and a lovely, understated punctuation.

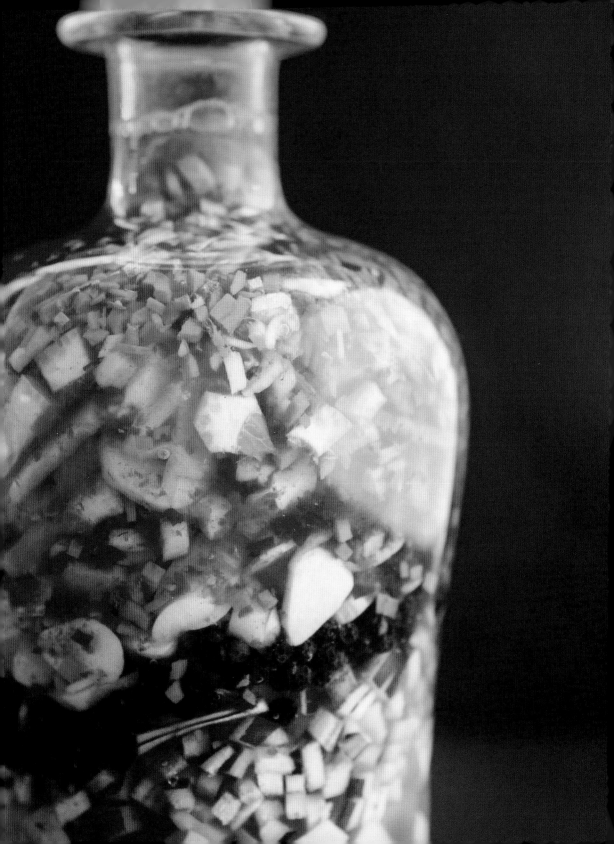

Fire Cider

FIRE CIDER IS A folk remedy to cure what ails you, popularized by Rosemary Gladstar. This is an infusion with an attitude—pungent, fiery, and sour. If you prefer it less pungent, you can make it with plenty of honey, as an oxymel. It's a remedy for colds, sinus congestion, and circulatory and digestive issues. For me, it works best if I take this in the first hour or two after I feel a cold coming on. There are many variations on the theme, where roots and herbs are steeped in the vinegar for a month or more, which draws out the healthful components. My husband, Christopher, and I have tasted some that are full of medicinal mushrooms and have a woodsy, earthy punch. This recipe is from our book *Fiery Ferments*. Drink it straight up, put it in warm water with honey or in cocktails, or cook with it.

YIELD
1½–2 quarts

¾ cup (168 g) horseradish root, peeled and finely diced

1–2 heads garlic, cloves peeled and minced

1 onion, diced

1 6-inch (15 cm) piece fresh ginger, diced

1 6-inch (15 cm) piece fresh turmeric root, diced

1 lemon, cut crosswise and sliced

2–3 tablespoons (14–21 g) peppercorns

6 tablespoons (51 g) fermented pepper mash (less if using habañero mash)

1½–2 quarts (1.4–1.9 L) raw, unfiltered, unpasteurized apple cider vinegar

1. Combine the prepared horseradish, garlic, onion, ginger, turmeric, lemon, peppercorns, and pepper mash in a sanitized jar. Pour in the vinegar until the jar is full. Stir. Use a plastic lid or place a piece of parchment paper, waxed cloth, or plastic wrap between the lid and the decoction to avoid corrosion. Tighten the lid and set aside for 4 to 5 weeks. Shake or stir the contents when you think about it.

2. Strain into a clean jar or bottle. Store in a cool, dark location, where it will keep for at least a year and usually much longer.

Q&A WITH ROSEMARY GLADSTAR

For anyone familiar with the modern American herbalist movement, Rosemary Gladstar needs no introduction. She is a world-renowned educator, activist, and entrepreneur and the founding director of Sage Mountain Herbal Retreat Center, the International Herb Symposium, and the New England Women's Herbal Conference. Gladstar is founding president of United Plant Savers, a nonprofit organization dedicated to the conservation and preservation of native American herbs. When I was a young homesteader, it was Rosemary's work that guided my herb gardens, my homespun tinctures, and my understanding of herbs. Years later, I was delighted to meet her through our publisher. Since then I have been honored to call her my friend and am honored that she lent her voice and knowledge to this book.

Q: *Vinegar has been used medicinally for thousands of years. As an herbalist, how do you see vinegar as part of the "medicine" available?*

A: Vinegar, especially raw apple cider vinegar, is a great tonic just by itself! Now, mix in some medicinal plants, and you have a superdrink. In many cultures around the world, vinegar-based drinks were enjoyed for health and healing purposes. Raw apple cider vinegar is a living substance teeming with healthy bacteria that are good for our gut. It is also high in an assortment of nutrients, including important vitamins and minerals. Although acidic and sour tasting, vinegar has an alkalizing effect in the body once digested.

Q: *Many herbs are infused into vinegars, mostly for culinary uses, but can you tell me how vinegar can be a powerful way to transmit the goodness of the herbs?*

A: Vinegar has the ability to absorb or draw out many of the plant's constituents, so it has been an important menstruum, or liquid, for making tinctures. It is especially good at extracting the water-soluble constituents, which include most of the vitamins, minerals, and other nutritional components of plants. Vinegar is also a natural preservative. Vinegar tinctures are generally thought to last for 8 to 12 months, but really, I've had vinegar tinctures that are still good after years of sitting in my pantry. Many other herbalists say the same.

Q: *How does using vinegar infusions to draw out the herb's constituents compare to alcohol or glycerin tinctures?*

A: Each of these substances—alcohol, vinegar, and glycerin—excels at drawing out different constituents of the plants. Without a doubt, alcohol is the strongest menstruum for making tinctures and has the longest shelf life. In my opinion, vinegar is the next strongest. While vinegar tinctures are never as potent as alcoholic tinctures, they are far better as nutritional supplements, are also excellent for children (especially when mixed with apple juice), and often advised for anyone averse to using alcoholic tinctures.

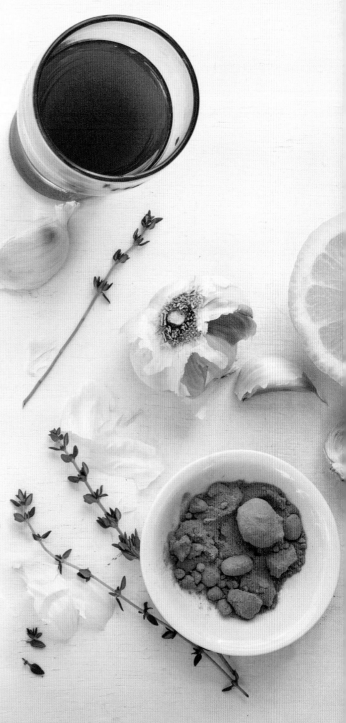

Q : *Let's talk about fire cider. You've brought this vinegar remedy to the forefront of herbal medicines. Can you share its story?*

A : Yes! Fire cider has become amazingly popular! Who would have ever thought? I concocted that first batch of fire cider in the herb school kitchen [the California School of Herbal Studies in Forestville, California] in the early 1980s. Of course, vinegar has been a popular home remedy for centuries, and there were many other vinegar recipes at the time. This one was built on others, as most recipes are. My goal that day working with my students was to create a tonic formula using commonly available kitchen ingredients that would warm us up from the inside out, that would taste good, and that would help to fend off colds and flus and other winter woes.

It definitely did that! When we tasted that first batch of fire cider after several weeks of steeping, we knew we had a winner. It was tasty, easy to make, inexpensive (just the cost of a quart of raw cider vinegar and common kitchen herbs, many of which could be grown in one's own garden), and it seemed to help boost one's immunity and keep one healthier if taken on a fairly regular basis. What wasn't to love?

Through the years, I taught hundreds of students how to make it, and they went on to teach their students. It was written about in books and magazine articles and was included in all of the early editions of my home-study course. Small companies were formed and started making fire cider as one of their products. It became one of those well-known—at least in the herbal circles—beloved and commonly shared herbal recipes.

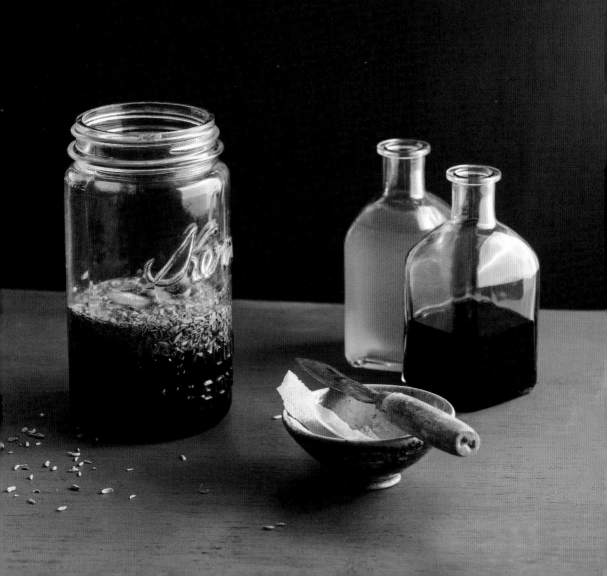

Vinegar Bitters

BITTER FOODS help activate the digestive system. When the bitterness hits our tongue, salivation immediately picks up production. This saliva helps break down carbs in our meal. It also stimulates the production of digestive enzymes and stimulates bile production, which our body uses to break down dietary fats. Because bitterness is lacking in our modern diets, our digestive systems don't work as well as they could. Adding bitters to our diet before meals can give our system a boost.

Traditionally, bitters have been made in alcoholic tinctures, but vinegar is becoming increasingly popular for digestive bitters. It is a natural choice because vinegar all by itself has many digestive benefits. This recipe uses everyday kitchen herbs, each chosen to stimulate and soothe digestion, making it easy and safe. We also dilute the straight vinegar with a little bit of thick balsamic, which is still curative, to take the edge off for folks who need a "spoonful of sugar to help the medicine go down." This vinegar also makes a delicious salad dressing. Feel free to prepare the full recipe with regular raw apple cider vinegar. Take ½ to 1 teaspoon at least 15 minutes before meals.

YIELD
about 1½ cups

Peel of 1 orange, sliced off the orange with minimal pith

4 tablespoons (24 g) fennel seed

2 tablespoons (24 g) dried dandelion root

1 tablespoon (5 g) diced fresh ginger

1 cup (237 mL) raw, unfiltered, unpasteurized apple cider vinegar, plus extra as needed

½ cup (118 mL) balsamic vinegar (or balsamic style, page 121)

1. Tear the orange peel into smaller pieces and combine with the fennel, dandelion root, and ginger in a sanitized pint jar.

2. Pour in enough of both kinds of vinegar to cover the herbs.

3. Cover tightly and let sit in a warm spot for 3 to 4 weeks.

4. Strain out the herbs. Bottle the vinegar and store in a cool, dark location, where it will keep for at least a year and usually much longer.

OXYMELS

An oxymel is simply vinegar and honey, two of human's earliest medicines, often enhanced by the addition of herbs. Ancient pharmacopeias have many oxymel-based recipes (like Honey Sekanjabin, page 244). You may have even unknowingly consumed an oxymel as a health drink: You can find it as a premixed drink in grocery stores, containing apple cider vinegar, cayenne, lemon, and honey diluted in water. Once you have made an oxymel, you can use it to dress fresh garden greens, drizzle it on toast, mix it into a little bubbly water for a refreshing pick-me-up, stir it into warm water for soothing relief, or take it straight up by the spoonful.

Make Your Own Oxymel

There are a number of ways to make an oxymel. It really depends on whether you want to infuse the herbs in the honey or the vinegar, or if you want to mix everything together and wait. See the Vinegar Reduction Infusion recipe on page 259 for an infused vinegar oxymel. As with all ancient recipes, the process for making oxymel is based on generations of makers handing down their practices all over the world. The ratios of honey to vinegar are also quite varied—from five parts honey to one part vinegar to the near opposite, three parts vinegar to one part honey. For these instructions, I split the difference, using half honey and half vinegar. You may want to start there and adjust to suit your tastes.

There is one rule: Don't heat your honey. You can heat and reduce your vinegar all you want, but keep your honey raw. Ancient wisdom warns against heating, and there are also some pretty compelling modern studies that show heating honey denatures the enzymes and creates a chemical that is thought to be a carcinogen.

Choose the herbs you want to use. There are many wonderful standard herbal formulas to strengthen or support your body that you can make into an oxymel. (And refer to the work of your favorite herbalist for more information on how to choose herbs that will work for you.)

HONEY CONSIDERATIONS

Have you ever stopped to consider honey? Our grocery store shelves are lined with honey jars, and little plastic packages of honey (or a combination of corn syrup and honey) often come with toast in cafés, so it is not surprising that most of us never think about how people used get honey. They would track and follow the bees back to their hives, where they would endure the stinging attacks to rob a bit of honey. Why? Because it is a remarkable substance—powerful and perfect in so many ways—delicious and healing, and it never goes bad. It is antibacterial and a complex combination of carbohydrates, proteins, phytochemicals, and antioxidants—a balanced diet for bees. It is their larder, and they work hard for it. One bee, capable of flying about 60 miles a day, will make only a half teaspoon of honey in her lifetime. Just imagine how many bee miles are in each quart of honey. When I first heard this, I became more conscious of my honey use, not that I used it indiscriminately, but I wanted to be sure my uses honored the substance that it is and the bees that made it. For me, herbal honeys and oxymels are some of the foods that fit beautifully into these self-imposed criteria.

All-in-One Oxymel

In this oxymel, everything is stirred together at the same time. This works well with honey that is still liquid. If your honey is thickening or crystallized, infuse herbs in vinegar for a couple of weeks and then add the strained warmed vinegar to the honey, as the thick honey can get stuck in the herbs, making it difficult to remove the herbs without wasting honey. In general, use one part dried herb to three or four parts vinegar and honey.

1. Fill a sanitized pint jar about one-quarter full of the selected and prepared herb (chopped as needed).

2. Fill the rest of the jar with equal parts vinegar and honey. The vinegar should be warmed to about 120°F/49°C—you don't want to cook the vinegar or overheat the honey—about 1½ cups (355 mL) of each. Add the warmed vinegar first and allow to cool a bit before adding the honey.

3. Stir well before sealing.

4. Place the jar on the counter but out of direct sunlight. Shake every few days to redistribute the herbs. Allow to infuse for at least 2 weeks.

5. Once infused, strain out the herbs or botanicals through a coffee filter or a few layers of cheesecloth. Toss the soaked herbs into the compost or, better yet, save to flavor a chutney or other condiment.

6. Store the oxymel in an airtight bottle or jar, with a glass and rubber-seal bail-type top or plastic lid that will not corrode over time. If you don't have either, place parchment paper, waxed cloth, or plastic wrap between the vinegar and lid.

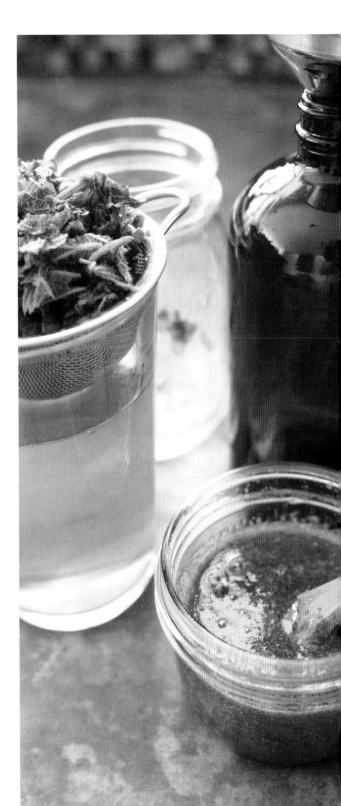

Nettle Oxymel

NETTLE MIGHT JUST BE my favorite herb. I look forward to the tender greens in early spring. We eat them, we ferment them in sauerkraut, and I infuse them in vinegar. Mineral-rich with iron, calcium, magnesium, silicone, and vitamins A, C, and D, they are also a powerful adaptogen herb—important for our adrenals and stress response. When fresh, they are also a natural antihistamine; fresh nettles used in vinegar preparations will retain this quality. Nettle oxymel is tasty in salad dressings or as a drinking tonic.

YIELD
about 2 cups

2 tablespoons (3 g) nettle seed

½ cup (170 g) raw honey

1½ cups (355 mL) vinegar of your choice

1½ cups (30 g) chopped fresh nettle, stems and leaves

1. Mix the nettle seed into the raw honey in a sanitized half-pint jar. Cover with the lid and tighten. Set aside.

2. Pour the vinegar into a stainless steel saucepan and heat over low heat to warm slightly, to about 135°F/57°C. Watch it carefully; you don't want to cook it at all. This is just to help get those enzymes to break down the nettle.

3. Finely chop the nettle, stems and all, and put in a pint jar.

4. Pour your warmed vinegar over the herbs. They should be completely covered. Stir them in to make sure they are submerged.

5. Screw on the jar lid, slipping a bit of parchment paper, waxed cloth, or plastic wrap between the jar and the metal lid to prevent corrosion of the lid.

6. Place the jars on your counter (but out of direct sunlight) so you remember to shake the vinegar jar every few days to redistribute the contents. Let it infuse for 2 weeks.

7. After 2 weeks, strain the nettle out of the vinegar. Line a strainer with a piece of butter muslin or fine-mesh cheesecloth and strain the mixture into a new sanitized jar. Squeeze the cloth to get all the liquid out. (Set the pickled herbs aside to refrigerate in a small jar for another use—salad dressing, garnish, you get the idea.)

8. Mix the strained vinegar with the seed honey. When thouroughly mixed, put in a storage jar with a noncorrosive lid. This will last indefinitely.

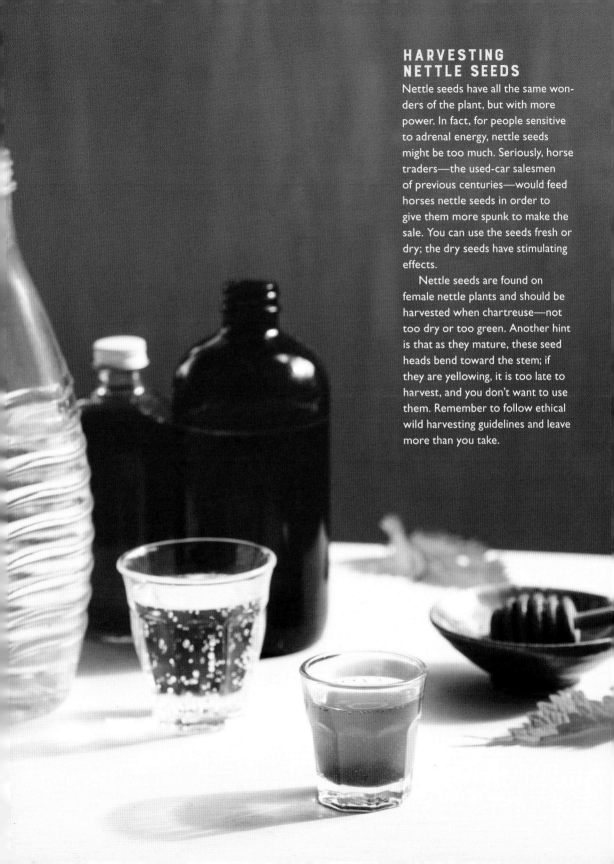

HARVESTING NETTLE SEEDS

Nettle seeds have all the same wonders of the plant, but with more power. In fact, for people sensitive to adrenal energy, nettle seeds might be too much. Seriously, horse traders—the used-car salesmen of previous centuries—would feed horses nettle seeds in order to give them more spunk to make the sale. You can use the seeds fresh or dry; the dry seeds have stimulating effects.

Nettle seeds are found on female nettle plants and should be harvested when chartreuse—not too dry or too green. Another hint is that as they mature, these seed heads bend toward the stem; if they are yellowing, it is too late to harvest, and you don't want to use them. Remember to follow ethical wild harvesting guidelines and leave more than you take.

APPENDICES
TROUBLESHOOTING

Slow Fermentation

Vinegar fermentation works best in temperatures that are warmer than the ambient temperature in most modern homes. The sweet spot is 77° to 86°F/ 25° to 30°C. If your temperatures are consistently lower than that, the ferment will take longer. This can be remedied by warming up the liquid, either by finding a warmer spot or submerging your vessel partway in a warm-water bath like that provided by an immersion circulator.

It could be that your raw starter vinegar or mother is no longer viable. If you suspect this is the case, you might leave it be and wait longer. Remember: Vinegar will begin over time without any starter.

If this doesn't work, it may be a lack of nutrients for the yeast or too much acidity. Either of these conditions can make it problematic for the bacteria to reproduce. Add a little bit of fruit juice to feed the yeast and reduce acidity.

Finally, if fermentation still doesn't begin, it could be that the base juice or alcohol contained sulfites or preservatives.

Vinegar Has a Film on Top that Isn't the Mother

When the mother is forming, it will be wispy thin, transparent, and the color of the base medium. If you smell closely, you might get a whiff of what smells like nail-polish remover (acetate). It will also hold together if you touch it gently. If this is the case, you can do a happy dance: Your vinegar is doing its thing.

If you have something that separates or breaks apart like cracking polar ice when touched, or that looks white or dusty (a bit like a moonscape with wrinkles and craters), then it is a yeast bloom. These yeasts (generally called kahm yeast) are harmless to you but can eventually cause the vinegar issues. For one, the yeast is a fungus. As it thrives, it can damage the acetic acid, taking the pH levels up instead

of down. This can also cause another fungus— mold—to get a foothold over time. Mold will spoil the vinegar.

Kahm yeast can be controlled. First, skim it off and start stirring daily to discourage growth. If it continues to be an issue, you can place the vinegar in a new container. Another effective strategy is to first skim it off or stir vigorously to knock it back, then treat the surface and the sides of the vessel with vodka or other 80 proof alcohol. Spritz a light mist on the surface and side walls any time you see this film, and it usually gives up. It is quite successful in most cases. Stop spritzing when it is no longer a problem. You will also want to make sure that the pH is at 4.0 or lower. If it isn't, add more raw vinegar to bring the pH within range, and make sure the temperature is at optimal range, too. Yeasts thrive at lower temperatures.

If you see mold, remove it immediately. Next, run the vinegar through a coffee filter. You may also want to pasteurize it by removing the mother, if you have one, and bringing the liquid to 140°F/60°C, holding it there for 30 minutes and then allowing it to cool. Rinse the mother off with cool water and set it aside in a jar with raw vinegar covering it. If you do this, you will need to add more starter and put the mother back on. Make sure that the pH

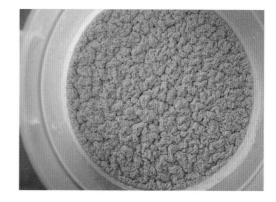

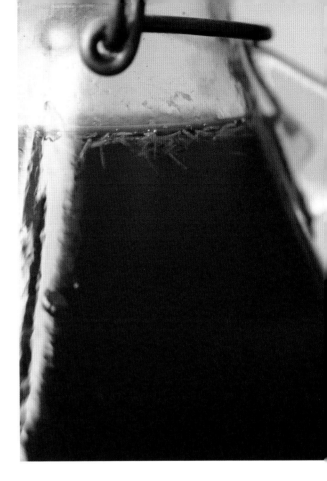

is at 4.0 or lower. If it isn't, add more raw vinegar. If you've pasteurized it, after it cools, make sure the temperature is within the optimal range.

Both kahm yeast and mold are fungi that are feeding off the vinegar. Prolonged periods with either of these surface layers will weaken the vinegar and prevent it from developing strong acidity.

Vinegar Mother Is Brown and Sinks

It's time to remove the mother. It's no longer alive. If you don't remove it, the vinegar will at some point smell and taste musty. Once you remove the mother, pour the vinegar through a coffee filter, which will help you avoid any mustiness. I found that one filter will accommodate 2 to 3 quarts (1.9 to 2.8 liters) of vinegar. Use a new filter for every few quarts, as I've found more times than I'd like to admit that pushing a filter for just a little more usually ends up with a blown-out filter—which means starting all over again.

Vinegar Smells like Nail-Polish Remover

This is not a fault; it's actually a good sign. It means the process is moving along, but just not done. This smell is the transitional step in the transformation taking place. Let me explain:

Alcohol (ethanol) + oxygen becomes acetaldehyde (the smell).

Acetaldehyde + oxygen becomes acetic acid and water = vinegar.

Vinegar Smells/Tastes Funky (like Sauerkraut)

This means that instead of developing acetic acid, your brew is turning sour due to lactic acid. I do not know of a fix for this. If there is a mother and it is fermenting, you can let it finish. The acetic acid may well kill the lactic acid bacteria, and over the course

of fermentation, it may right itself. There may be lingering lactic sourness, but this is not harmful.

Vinegar Eels

Vinegar eels (*Turbatrix acei*) sound worse than they are. They are nematodes that feed off the mother and look like little worms wiggling around in the vinegar. They are unappetizing for sure but harmless and not parasitic. So if you ingest them, they will not do anything besides pass innocuously right on through your digestive system. They will eventually degrade the health of the mother, though, as they feed on the beneficial microbes.

Vinegar eels can be seen with the naked eye but can go unnoticed for quite some time as the populations start small. If you suspect eels, take your vinegar (assuming it is in a clear jar) into a dark room and shine a flashlight through the side. If your fermentation is in a barrel or ceramic vessel, shine the light through the top. You will see them wriggle toward the light.

If you discover vinegars eels, you should toss the infected mother into the compost. You will never get a clean batch from that mother again. You can filter the vinegar with a coffee filter, then consume it—just don't use this vinegar to start new batches. If you are using a wooden barrel to age your vinegar, chances are that you will not be able to use that container again either without getting eels. If you have made multiple batches, check them all for infestation, and if present, you will need to start over with everything. Not all is lost, though, if you own fish: It turns out the eels are great fish food (some folks breed them for just that purpose).

How do you end up with eels? Open vinegar brews can be susceptible, or the nematodes may come in from a raw commercial vinegar. It happens to the big guys, too—they just strain them out. All that said, eels are not a given. I have been making open vinegars, and vinegars started with commercial vinegars, for nine years and have never experienced eels.

Overoxidation

The process of making vinegar is oxidation, but your vinegar can also *over*oxidize. If your vinegar loses acidity and tastes watery, it has overoxidized. This is when the bacteria run out of alcohol, but instead of dying without that food source, they are capable of metabolizing the acid they just created and leaving only water and carbon dioxide.

This is a problem that home makers can experience when leaving their vinegar open for long periods (who hasn't forgotten a fermentation project?) or storing raw vinegar with live bacteria in a container that isn't airtight. This is usually a gradual deterioration, but you will notice it. You might see color changes, like a browning that appears near the top and grows downward. There may be no color change but the pizzazz and pop of the acidic flavor and esters are gone. You can check any vinegar you suspect has overoxidized with pH strips; you want the pH to stay below 4.0. As ever, the percent acid is a more difficult measurement. A vinegar that loses acidity is no longer bulletproof. Throw away anything that is watery, or if you are in doubt. Other microbes—fungi, yeasts, and/or lactic acid bacteria—will destroy acetic acid when it is diluted by oxidation.

Overoxidation can be avoided with airtight storage, which includes no headspace in the vessel. Be mindful of this when your bottle of homemade vinegar is getting low: Simply transfer the vinegar to a smaller bottle to minimize that empty air space. Alternatively, pasteurize the vinegar before storage.

If you suspect a small amount of oxidation and the vinegar is weak but vibrant, it is possible to add a small amount of high-proof alcohol to bring it back into balance. I don't have specific instructions for this—it's just something I have experimented with—but it has worked for me when the vinegar isn't too far gone. To verify that the added alcohol has corrected the issue, test the vinegar and make sure the pH is still below 4.0. The vinegar should become strong and bright. If this doesn't happen, your vinegar is too far gone.

A PRIMER ON GROWING KOJI

Each of the recipes in this book can be made with koji rice that is inoculated and ready to go. (See Resources for purchasing options, page 285.) This section is meant to give you enough knowledge to get started with koji and use it for brewing and vinegar making, but be warned: Koji has a reputation of turning into an addicting hobby, with makers looking around thinking "I wonder what will happen if I grow koji on _____?" Or, simply, "What can I kojify next?" You have been warned! If you want to dive deeper into the how to and potential of working with koji, Christopher and I delve into the finer points in the book *Miso, Tempeh, Natto & Other Tasty Ferments*.

Koji can seem intimidating; I know this well. I was apprehensive for longer than I care to admit. Later, I realized that the most overwhelming part is actually pretty simple—getting past my own mind, overthinking the whole thing. The second issue is getting the incubation system dialed in. I try to remind people that nothing I teach is new or high tech; people have been doing these things to transform food with microbes for thousands of years, with very little in the way of equipment. They just did it and we can, too.

A Quick Guide to Incubating Koji

When working with koji, you want to keep your space, your implements, and your hands clean. Remember that there are many other (unwelcome) microbes out there, like bread mold and *Bacillus subtilis*, that would welcome the opportunity to join the party. This is not to say that you need to drive yourself crazy with sterilization; you just want to make sure your work area is clean. As an extra measure, I sanitize all the utensils I will be using by one of three methods: misting a bit of 80 proof alcohol (40 percent alcohol) or brewing sanitizer across the surface and air-drying; pouring boiling water over the surface and keeping it there for at least 30 seconds and then air-drying; or using the sanitation cycle of our dishwasher. You can also sanitize glass casserole dishes or jars by washing them in hot, soapy water and putting them in a microwave for 45 seconds or until dry.

Koji grains are traditionally steamed, which renders them al dente, with the individual kernels easily separated. They will feel slightly rubbery. When steamed, the grains are more likely to give you a koji that resembles what you might purchase, with separated grains that have a light dusting of mycelium.

YELLOW, WHITE, AND BLACK

These are the colors used to describe members of the *Aspergillus* species used in brewing and food production in Japan. Yellow, white, and black refer to the color of the spores of these different species of *Aspergillus*. Yellow koji (*Aspergillus oryzae*) is the most common—it is used in miso, sake, and soy sauces. It is a little more temperamental and requires lower temperatures than black. It does not produce citric acid at all. It is characterized by its beguiling scent. White koji (also *Aspergillus kawachi*) is a mutation of black, easier to grow, and its enzymes are strong amylase producers, which results in a lot of released sugar. It is most often used to produce shochu, a Japanese distilled spirit.

Black koji (*Aspergillus luchenis* var. *awarmori*) is said to extract flavor characteristics of the base ingredient better, resulting in more aromas, but the superpower in vinegar making is that it creates citric acid; it's great to begin the vinegar making process with some nice acidity.

I've found that cooking the grains in a rice cooker or in a pot also works, so long as the cooked grains are not soggy but al dente. This cooking method creates more of a soft, matted koji, where the individual grains are hard to distinguish.

Whole grains with their hard casings intact are difficult for the hyphae (koji roots) to penetrate, so they must be somehow broken open. This is why you will often see white rice or pearled barley as common substrates. However, given one doesn't want to be limited by this, all you have to do is make sure you handle or cook the grains in a way that breaks open the shell. This can be done with cooking or physically cracking the grains.

When preparing grains that are in a meal form, like cornmeal, for koji, you need to cook it in a way that cooks and penetrates the grain with moisture without getting it soggy or sticky. The best way I have found to do this is to take the meal and put it into a bag for vacuum sealing food. For example, with cornmeal, place about 2 cups of cornmeal in a bag that has been cut to accommodate this meal and add ½ to ¾ cup (118 to 177 mL) water. You will add the water a little at a time to the bag and mix thoroughly until you have an even moisture. It should be a crumbly consistency in the way a pie crust dough is. Vacuum seal the bag, then cook in a large pot of water, or sous vide, that you keep between 160° and 180°F/71° and 82°C for two hours. When the cornmeal is cooked, you crumble it up into your casserole dish and proceed with inoculation and incubation, as you would with any whole grain.

Inoculation

Place the cooked substrate into a casserole dish or tray or onto butter muslin. Break up the lumps and spread it out so steam can escape. Allow the substrate to cool to around 110°F/43°C.

As the substrate cools, toast flour in a dry pan over medium heat until lightly browned, to sterilize.

This can be all-purpose flour, rice flour, tapioca flour, even cornstarch—choose your preference. The goal is to disperse the spores and give them easy food to get started. Sterilizing the flour ensures that the koji mold will not have to compete with other microbes in the early stages of its growth.

Add the spores to the cool toasted flour.

Sprinkle half of the koji-flour starter into the substrate and mix. The substrate will take on a light olive green coating. Add the rest of the starter and mix until you are confident that your substrate is evenly coated.

Aspergillus likes a bit of humidity, so at this point you may need to cover your fermentation tray. Your incubation method will determine what type of covering will work best. It may be a damp, clean cotton cloth in a proofing box, an oven, or another system that produces dry heat. In a dehydrator, the airflow is so dry that you will want to use plastic wrap poked with a couple of diagonally opposite holes at the ends of the tray to allow airflow. If you are using a water-bath incubator, you won't need to cover the tray, just the tub.

CAUTION: *It is important that you avoid inhaling the spores.* The spores can clump in your lungs, where they cannot be expelled, making you sick. One strategy to avoid airborne spores is to carefully measure the spores into a small bowl, then gently add the flour on top; the flour will weigh down the spores when you stir them. If you have a compromised immune system, wear a dust mask at all times when working with spores.

Incubation

This is the part of the fermentation that can feel the most intimidating.

It's true that koji does need specific conditions to grow. Koji thrives in a similar environment to what we humans prefer, if maybe a little on the warmer side. To grow and metabolize, koji likes to be between 80° and 95°F/27° and 35°C. The exception is *Aspergillus luchenis,* or black koji. It should be incubated at 104°F/40°C for the first 12 hours.

For small batches of koji, I have found an immersion circulator to be ideal. I set the water temperature at 88°F/31°C and don't have to monitor the internal temperature of the koji. A bread proofing box is my second favorite, as the temperature setting, in my experience, is very responsive and on target. And while you still have to monitor the internal temps of the koji, you aren't dealing with the drying air of a dehydrator. (A caution: If you try to fit too many trays in a proofing box, you may lose some airflow, and your koji may not do well.)

The first few times you make koji, be prepared to babysit it for a few days. Like anything that's alive, it doesn't follow a mechanical clock. While it is generally pretty consistent, you'll likely encounter some batches that follow a different schedule. Be sure to observe, smell, and touch as needed to make sure you are on track. Once you get into the groove of making it and know the particulars of your incubation equipment and technique, the process becomes much easier.

THE FIRST 12 TO 18 HOURS, keep it at 90°F/32°C. Keep the internal temperature between 80° and 95°F/27° and 35°C. Once the koji starts to metabolize, it keeps itself warm; in fact, it generates a lot of heat, which must be dissipated. Above 95°F/35°C, it will overheat, which is perhaps the most common reason for failure.

THROUGHOUT THE PROCESS, you must dissipate enough heat to prevent the koji from overheating and self-destructing. Temperature can be lowered, and the koji can be stirred to gently break up the clumps to keep it from overheating. You can make furrows in the bed, which offers more surface area for dispersing heat.

After 18 to 24 hours, you will notice a fuzzy white coating on your substrate. It will start to have a pleasant, yeasty, floral, mushroomy, distinctly sweet smell.

After 30 to 50 hours, the koji will be done. The great variation in incubation time depends on substrate. Koji is finished when it is cottony and fuzzy and almost looks a little blurry, as if your eyes aren't quite focusing. If the koji has begun to produce spores, it will also have fuzzy patches of yellow-green; you want to stop incubating as soon as you see this. Put it in the fridge, sealed, until ready to use.

Use soon. The fresher the koji, the better it is for sugars. When making amazake or sake for vinegar, use it as soon as possible.

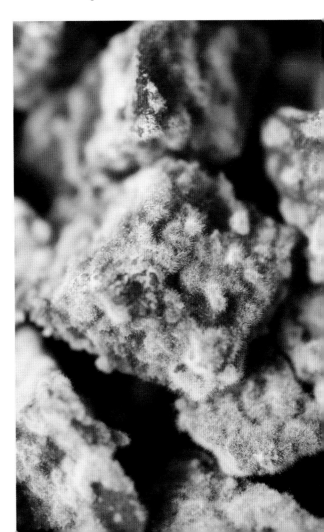

How to Grow Koji

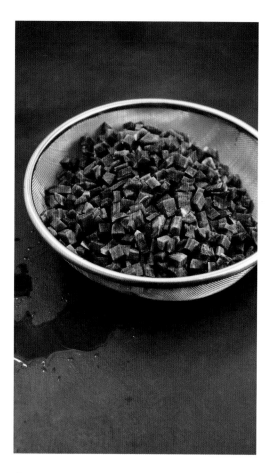

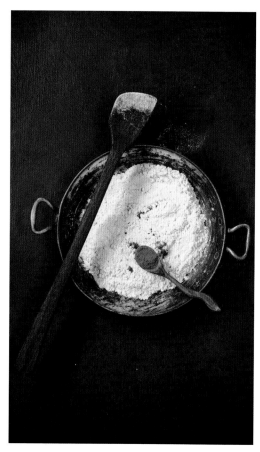

1. Sanitize your tools and work surface before getting started. Dice and cook sweet potatoes until al dente. Put in a colander to drain and allow the steam to dissipate, so that the outside of the pieces dry.

2. While the potatoes are cooking, toast all-purpose wheat flour or rice flour in a small skillet over medium heat to sterilize it. When the flour is cool, stir it into a bowl with the koji spores. Take care. The spores are very light and will want to float away.

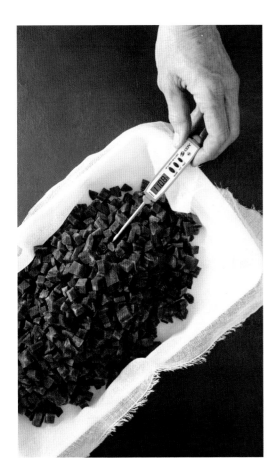

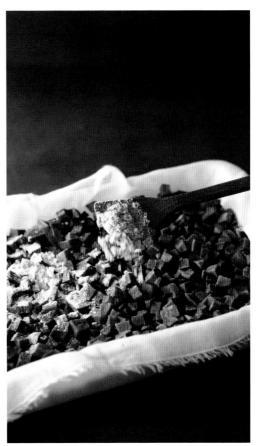

3. Spread the potatoes out in a glass casserole dish lined with a piece of cheesecloth and cool to 110°F/43 °C.

4. Sprinkle half of the koji-flour mixture on the potatoes.

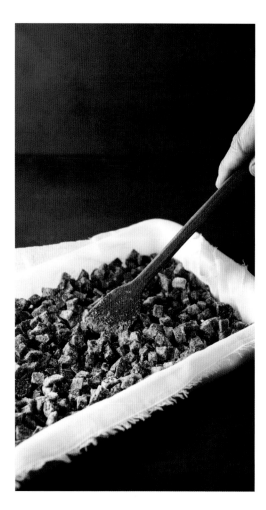

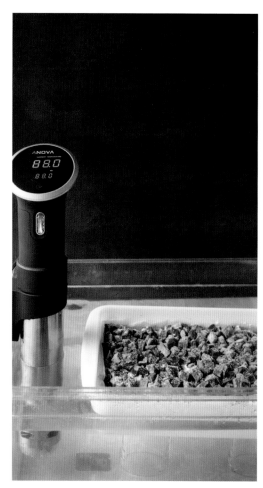

5. Fold in the koji gently to evenly disperse the spores, gently breaking up clumps as you go. Then sprinkle on the rest of the koji-flour mixture and gently stir again.

6. Place the dish in a sous vide water bath and set to 104°F/40°C for *Aspergillus luchensis* or 88°F/31°C for *A. oryzae*. Be sure to tuck your cheesecloth inside the dish. If you don't, it will wick water into the dish, drowning the koji.

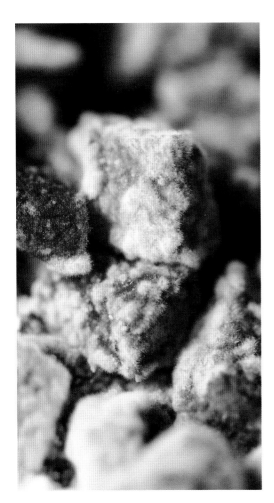

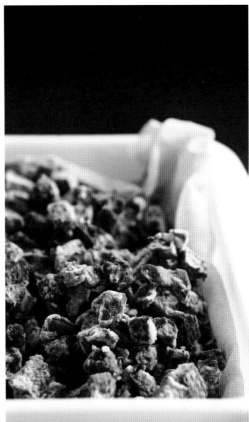

7. After 24 hours, the koji will smell faintly aromatic in a sweet, floral, mushroomy way. The surface will appear to have the beginning blush of a soft white covering. It will be partly bound together. Check the temperature again to make sure it is in the correct range.

8. When finished, the koji will have a cottony appearance, and some pieces may be knit together in a mycelial mat. Transfer to a widemouthed jar, seal with an airtight lid, and refrigerate.

ENDNOTES

1   Stuckey, 2012.

2   Štornik et al., 2016.

3   Yan, 2018.

4   Boyer, 2004.

5   Shahidi et al., 2008.

6   Schaeffer et al., 2016

7   Pozo et al., 2018

8   Kuanyshev et al., 2017.

9   Norihiko et al., 2003.

10   Sengun and Karabiyikli, 2011

11   Johnston et al., 2004

12   Johnston et al., 2004.

CITATIONS

Boyer J, RH Liu. "Apple Phytochemicals and Their Health Benefits." *Nutrition Journal* 3, no. 5 (2004): 1475–2891 :5.

Fabian, Fredrick W. "Honey Vinegar." Michigan State College of Agriculture and Applied Science, 1935. Extension Bulletin 149. archive.lib.msu.edu/DMC/Ag.%20Ext.%202007-Chelsie/PDF/e149.pdf

Johnston CS, CM Kim, AJ Buller. "Vinegar Improves Insulin Sensitivity to a High-Carbohydrate Meal in Subjects with Insulin Resistance or Type 2 Diabetes." *Diabetes Care* 27, no. 1 (2004): 281–282.2.

Kuanyshev N, GM Adamo, D Porro, P Branduardi. "The Spoilage Yeast *Zygosaccharomyces bailii*: Foe or Friend?" *Yeast* 34, no. 9 (2017): 359–370.

Norihiko, Terahara, Toshiro Matsui, Keiichi Fukui, Kazusato Matsugano, Koichi Sugita, and Kiyoshi Matsumoto. "Caffeoylsophorose in a Red Vinegar Produced through Fermentation with Purple Sweet Potato." *Journal of Agricultural and Food Chemistry* 51, no. 9 (2003): 2539–2543.

Pozo MI, J Bartlewicz, A van Oystaeyen. "Surviving in the Absence of Flowers: Do Nectar Yeasts Rely on Overwintering Bumblebee Queens to Complete Their Annual Life Cycle?" *FEMS Microbiol Ecology* 94, no. 12 (2018): 10.

Schaeffer, Robert N., et al. "Consequences of a Nectar Yeast for Pollinator Preference and Performance." *Functional Ecology* 31, no. 3 (2016): 613–621.

Sengun, Ilkin, Seniz Karabiyikli. "Importance of acetic acid bacteria in food industry." *Food Control* 22, no. 5 (2011): 647–656.

Shahidi F, J McDonald, A Chandrasekara, Y Zhong. "Phytochemicals of Foods, Beverages, and Fruit Vinegars: Chemistry and Health Effects." *Asia Pacific Journal of Clinical Nutrition* 17, Supp; 1, no. 1 (2008): 380–382.

Štornik A, B Skok, J Trček. "Comparison of Cultivable Acetic Acid Bacterial Microbiota in Organic and Conventional Apple Cider Vinegar." *Food Technology & Biotechnology* 54, no. 1 (2016): 113–119.

Stuckey, Barb. *Taste: Surprising Stories and Science about Why Food Tastes Good*. Atria, 2012.

Yan JW, et al. "The Aroma Volatile Repertoire in Strawberry Fruit: A Review." *Journal of the Science of Food and Agriculture* 98, no. 12 (2018): 4395–4402.

RESOURCES

The Eternal Condiment

You could spend hours getting lost and going down fascinating rabbit holes on Reginald Smith's blog, Supreme Vinegar.

https://supremevinegar.com/the-eternal-condiment -vinegar-blog/

FARMcurious

This urban homestead supply has the most beautiful wooden continuous-brew vinegar barrel. They also sell mothers and a starter kit.

www.farmcurious.com

Home Brew Supply

There are many online resources for converting degrees Brix to specific gravity and vice versa. This link is a handy online calculator that will do both.

https://homebrewsupply.com/brix-conversion -calculator

Kombucha Kamp

This site has many types of brewing pots and vessels. It also has jackets and stick-on thermometers, which can be handy for keeping things warm enough.

www.kombuchakamp.com

Lady Jayne's Alchemy

Jori Jayne Emde offers bespoke orders, consulting, and online classes through her website. She has a lot of knowledge to share if you want to continue your journey. (See the profile on page 182.)

www.ladyjaynesalchemy.com

Midwest Supplies

Complete brewing supplies. Their physical store is in Minneapolis, Minnesota.

www.midwestsupplies.com

USDA ARS Culture Collection (NRRL)

The ARS Culture Collection is one of the largest public collections of microorganisms in the world, containing approximately 98,000 isolates of bacteria and fungi. It's a treasure trove for the fermenter. This was my source of *Kluyveromyces marxianus* for whey vinegar.

https://nrrl.ncaur.usda.gov

ARTISAN MAKERS

American Vinegar Works

Using American craft ciders, wines, and beers, this vinegar company in Lowell, Massachusetts, uses traditional slow brewing methods.

www.americanvinegarworks.com

George Paul Vinegar

Beautiful, handcrafted vinegars made on a family farm in the Sandhills of Nebraska.

www.georgepaulvinegar.com

Hani Honey Company

Family run, this Florida honey company is going above and beyond to work with the bees and the plants that are available locally. Their honey is over the top amazing. (See the profile on page 208.)

www.hanihoneycompany.com

Keepwell Vinegar

The team behind Keepwell describes themselves as two pastry chefs who decided to push sugar in a different way. This small vinegar company sources the best local ingredients it can, to create unparalleled flavor.

www.keepwellvinegar.com

Madhouse Vinegar Co.

A small-batch maker with a flagship line and unique seasonal offerings. (See the profile on page 197.)

www.goodvinegar.com

McClary Bros.

These drinking vinegars are made with local, organic ingredients and are delicious.

www.mcclarybros.com

Slide Ridge

Based in Utah, this family-run company ranks beekeeping and healthy bees as its number one priority. The product they make to showcase their honey is a Honey Wine Vinegar.

www.slideridge.com

Supreme Vinegar

Reginald Smith's vinegar works has a delightful selection of raw vinegar and various types of vinegar mothers to get you started. (See the profile on page 19.)

www.supremevinegar.com

Traditional Aceto Balsamico of Monticello

The Darlands make true Aceto Balsamico in New Mexico. (See the profile on page 112.)

www.organicbalsamic.com

KOJI SPORES

Fermentationculture.eu

Koji spores and koji rice

www.fermentationculture.eu

GEM Cultures

They carry the biggest variety of koji spores, as well as inoculated rice and barley, natto spores, and other milk and grain cultures, including sourdough.

www.gemcultures.com

Higuchi Moyashi

This long-time family-run company has a wide variety of different, harder-to-find koji strains.

www.higuchi-m.co.jp/english/index.html

South River Miso Company

South River Miso carries a wonderful selection of miso and is a good resource for US-made organic brown rice koji.

www.southrivermiso.com

SUGGESTED READING

BOOKS ABOUT MAKING VINEGAR

Advances in Vinegar Production **by Dr. Argyro Bekatorou**

This is a textbook-style book for those who are looking for a deep dive into the science.

The Artisanal Vinegar Maker's Handbook **by Bettina Malle and Helge Schmickl**

The authors give detailed instructions for setting up a vinegar generator system.

Brew Beer Like a Yeti **or** *Make Mead Like a Viking* **both by Jereme Zimmermann**

These are great resources for anyone who wants to brew their own ale and beer or mead with more traditional methods.

Koji Alchemy **by Jeremy Umansky and Rich Shih**

This is a deep dive into many aspects of koji, including how it's used for making vinegar.

Kombucha, Kefir, and Beyond **by Alex Lewin and Raquel Guajardo**

I love this book for its approachability. It has many easy recipes for quick fermented beverages. It has some vinegar recipes as well.

The Noma Guide to Fermentation **by David Zilber and Rene Redzepi**

Making vinegar with spirits is discussed at length.

Sacred and Herbal Healing Beers **by Stephen Harrod Buhner**

An interesting and useful book in understanding the history of brews, especially those made with botanicals.

Vinegar: The User-Friendly Standard Text Reference & Guide to Appreciating, Making, and Enjoying Vinegar **by Lawrence J. Diggs**

This book got many recent amateur and artisan vinegar makers started.

The Wildcrafted Brewer **by Pascal Baudar**

Baudar outlines many wild ingredient recipes that can easily become vinegar.

BOOKS THAT USE VINEGAR IN RECIPES

Acid Trip by Michael Harlan Turkell
A fun read: This jaunt through some of the world's finest vinegars with recipes is less of a recipe book, but I have been delighted by the ones I tried.

Fire Cider by Rosemary Gladstar and Friends
101 recipes from herbalists all over the country for making vinegar-based fire cider. It also features great discussions and ideas for using vinegar as medicine in folk remedies.

House of Vinegar by Jonathan Sawyer
A chef's look at vinegar in his kitchen. Some recipes for vinegar, but mostly a cookbook using vinegar.

The Vinegar Cupboard by Angela Clutton
A wonderful read on many traditional vinegars and how to use them. There aren't recipes for making vinegar but many ideas for ways to use unique vinegars.

Vinegar Revival by Harry Rosenblum
This approachable love letter to vinegar includes some vinegar making and a lot of great recipes for using vinegar.

BOOKS WITH A HISTORICAL FOCUS, FOR CONTEXT AND IDEAS

The Drunken Botanist by Amy Stewart
As we find ourselves looking more to the plants around us, this is a fascinating read on some of the plants that have played roles in our beverages.

Vinegar, the Eternal Condiment by Reginald Smith
This is the story of vinegar. It is a well-researched look at the history and how the science and business of vinegar developed throughout the world.

ACKNOWLEDGMENTS

I AM ETERNALLY GRATEFUL TO YOU, my readers, who have come along with me on one fermentation journey after another. Without you, this book would not be out in the world celebrating the sour work of acetic bacteria. And while we're speaking of microbes, I must thank that silent powerful work of the microbes that transform. These small players show up by the millions and do the job. Put your hands together for vinegar's team—yeast and acetic bacteria.

I am indebted to all vinegar makers, past and present, in all the regions of the world, who have understood the alchemy of an acid that has preserved, protected, and made our lives a little tastier with its sour punch.

I am always touched beyond words when people share their fermentation journeys with me. In some cases they share more—ideas, recipes, or, in the case of Janine Parr, a box of fresh dates to experiment with. Thank you, Janine, for your role in this book.

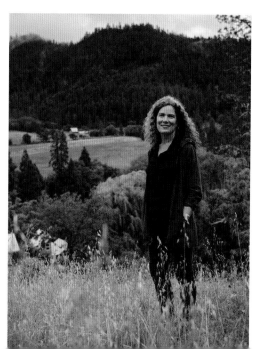

A book does not come into being without many mentors who patiently answer questions and talk through processes and projects. I am in awe of all the research Reginald Smith has done over the years and cannot thank him enough for his generosity in sharing this expertise. I am grateful to Steve Darland for taking the time to make sure I understood the beautiful alchemy that creates aceto balsamico in both process and flavor. I had wonderful conversations with Michael Harlan Turkell, Jori Jayne Emde, Jennifer Holmes, Richard Stewart, Jitti Chaithiraphant, Rosemary Gladstar, Mike Bowman, Jeremy Umansky, Martin James, Raquel Guarjardo, Antonio De Valle, Ken Fornataro, and Mara Jane King. I am grateful to each of you for guidance in helping me continue to learn.

I have a deep gratitude for the team at Storey, who can make an idea a reality. There are so many of you that touch the book both before and after it is born. I am appreciative, truly, of each of you and your work. Anastasia Whalen, here we go again! The idea for this book did not come from me; instead I must thank Sarah Guare, for it only came about because she said my vinegar chapter in *The Big Book of Cidermaking* was too large. Carleen Madigan, it has been a pleasure. Thank you for shaping the book and for the cheery emails, even when I was feeling salty. This book and its cover are absolutely beautiful thanks to the vision of Carolyn Eckert, and thanks to Carmen Troesser's magic behind the camera, with the help of Marcus J. Schwab.

I am humbled by my family's encouragement and willingness to keep tasting. And there may not be a big enough thank you to Christopher for cleaning up all the messes, and for his undying support and belief in what we do.

INDEX

Page numbers in *italics* indicate photos.

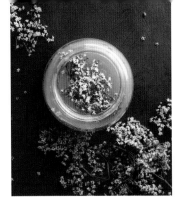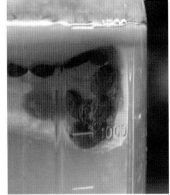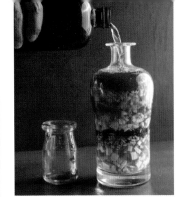

TECHNIQUES

RECIPES

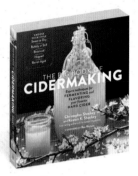
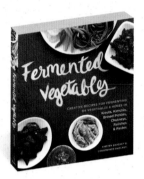
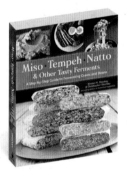
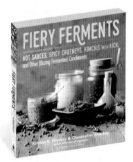